Diabetes?
No thanks!

Diabetes?
No thanks!

Lars-Erik Litsfeldt

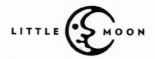

Published by Little Moon Publishing Ltd.,
3rd floor Premier House
12-13 Hatton Garden
London EC1N 8AN
UNITED KINGDOM

www.littlemoonpublishing.com

ISBN 978-1-908018-01-4

Text copyright Lars-Erik Litsfeldt © 2011

First English edition © 2011
Translated from Swedish by Janis Abens
Based upon the Swedish edition "*Diabetes? Nej tack!*",
first published by Optimal förlag, Sweden 2010.
This book is published by agreement with LCHF Sweden AB.
Designed in Norway
Printed by Nørhaven in Denmark
Cover design by Espen Pedersen, Norway

At what point does
being overweight become a disease,
and must we really develop diabetes
before we are prescribed a diet
that will prevent it?

Table of Contents

Swedish medical authorities have
confirmed that THE SCANDINAVIAN DIET,
as a treatment for obesity and diabetes,
is consistent with current scientific
understanding and proven experience.
For those of you longing to eat real food
again, wait no longer. Go for it and start
enjoying your new life!

My story

In January 2001 I was diagnosed with type 2 diabetes. The year before, I had started to drink more and more water. It was a gradual increase, and by the New Year, I had begun to keep a water bottle on my night table for use when I woke up. I was constantly trudging between the toilet and the kitchen tap. My HbAlc level – a kind of blood sugar measurement based on levels during the past few months – was determined to be 12.5.

Compare that to a normal level, which should be between 3.3 and 5.0. My blood sugar at that particular moment was 28, or about four to five times higher than it should have been.

I guess I was an "average" diabetic. I was overweight, hardly ever exercised, had slightly elevated blood pressure and had a family history of diabetes. When I saw my doctor and got my diagnosis, I was also given a prescription for medication and a few brochures about diabetes. I couldn't read all of them all the way through, but some of them were not that depressing.

I'll never forget the first morning I took my medication. I was to take a pill that would kickstart my pancreas and secrete insulin into my body. The basic idea was that the medication would quickly reduce the increased blood sugar levels

I would experience after breakfast. According to the brochures, that would be porridge and whole wheat bread. After finishing half of my porridge, I began to shiver and broke into a cold sweat. The medication had begun to work. I dragged myself to the refrigerator where I fumbled with a bottle of juice before managing to swallow a couple of swigs. I then lay down and began to feel how the shivering and cold sweat went away. After checking with the Swedish National Medical Information Centre, I received a comforting reply. I wasn't suffering from extremely low blood sugar, just an unexpectedly rapid decrease, from 20 to 15 within a few minutes.

That was great news, as I didn't want this to happen every morning. After a while, my blood sugar should stabilise at reasonable levels, and the rapid decrease wouldn't be as dramatic.

A week later, I met with a nurse and a nutritional physiologist. I was taught the importance of not eating any white bread. I was also told to be careful with mashed potatoes. Rice was bad as well, especially jasmine rice, which, naturally, was my favourite sort. Apparently, I could now eat nothing but whole wheat bread and vegetables – in any case, that's how it seemed. I was told that, from now on, I was obliged to eat the way other people *should* eat. I came to the conclusion that the easiest way to figure out what was okay to eat was: "If I like it, it's not good for me". As with most diabetics, it would also be helpful for me to lose some weight, which, of course, meant avoiding fatty foods. I was to choose the low-fat alternative whenever possible. Finally, I was ordered to exercise more.

About 10 months later – on a Thursday in the middle of

November – I suffered a minor heart attack. Heart attacks are not uncommon when one has diabetes. The basic "concept" is that it's not the actual diabetes that is life-threatening, but rather the various consequences of being a diabetic. Blood vessels and nerves are injured by all the sugar that's constantly circulating in the body. The artery walls deteriorate and blood clots can happen more easily. I was following my diet strictly and exercising every day, but this was apparently not helping.

A bit more than a year after I was diagnosed with diabetes, I had successfully reduced my HbAlc- level to 5.8 – in other words, barely higher than the levels of healthy people. On the other hand, my attempts at losing weight left quite a bit to be desired. I had to work on getting that weight down, and the blood sugar also, if possible. The only question was: how? I was really trying. I had reduced my fat intake and was eating even more vegetables, but I was still failing to lose weight or reduce my blood sugar level.

Foreword by the author

Several years have passed since I became interested in the effects of food on the human body. When I published my first book "Fettskrämd" ("Fear of Fat"), it was regarded as quite unconventional. During the manuscript phase, many publishers considered it "unsellable". A journalist who reviewed the book would always include a "fact column" where the so-called "experts" presented the "correct" facts. Every one of the facts contradicted the message in my book. I don't see those fact columns any longer. Actually, I've even seen health care professionals tout the advantages of the type of diet I advocate as their last word in diet articles.

There should certainly be room for a book specifically addressing diabetics. Books currently available for diabetics don't contain anything new. They're all about being careful with sugar and fat, providing a few recipes that are guaranteed to elevate a diabetic's blood sugar.

This book takes diabetes treatment another step forward, and it is different from other books about the treatment of this disease. The content of this book aims instead to help diabetics slow down progression of the disease as much as possible. It's about not raising blood sugar any more than necessary. Many people who take the contents of this book to heart will also improve their health dramatically.

I don't believe in repeating rules over and over to convince people. In order to succeed in sticking to a dietary model, we must first understand what happens in our bodies when we eat. Many people also have blind faith in the statements made by medical professionals, without even considering if they have the authority to make them. That's why much of this book aims to explain the mechanisms behind the poor level of diabetes treatment. After having read this book, other diabetes brochures and books you read will fill you with dismay because you will understand why the advice they provide is bad for you.

Introduction

Obviously, I have no idea who you are, sitting there with this book in your hand, but you probably have diabetes. Maybe someone who cares about you gave you the book. Or maybe you bought it yourself because you want to change your life.

Perhaps you've just found out that you have diabetes? If so, this news probably surprised you. In a matter of minutes you went from not feeling well, to being seriously ill. Your body feels exactly the same as the minute before you were told, but now you're ill. Really ill. You have discovered that you now need to prick your finger several times a day to check your blood sugar.

Maybe you've found out that you need to watch what you eat. Nevertheless, you're uncomfortable with the new situation. That's what I felt, anyway, when I found out I had become a type 2 diabetic. A multitude of questions popped into my head: What should I eat? Will I die soon? Will I need a membership card at the diabetes clinic? How often do diabetics have their feet amputated? What will happen to my vision!? Will I become a blind vegetable with no feet? How bad is my condition on a scale of 1 to 10? Maybe it's not that bad, or am

I deathly ill? How can I find out? Is it irreversible? Is there anything anyone can do to help? Is it like a snake pit, where I'll spend the rest of my life? Will I be able to climb out?

After the hospital visit during which I discovered that I really was a diabetic, they gave me some brochures that explained this diabetes thing. I was also told that I had to learn to eat healthily. The doctor told me that from now on, I MUST eat the way other people SHOULD eat. These were depressing words, indeed. Well, it's supposed to be good for me, but how good does it taste? I was presented with pictures of the plate model, food circles and pyramids and all that stuff, and it did not look appealing. At least, I didn't think so. But from now on, I would be eating low-fat, with lots of whole grain bread and plenty of pasta. I'd always choose the low-fat alternative because the others were dangerous. More than half of my food would be carbohydrates. I found out that my illness would worsen with time, even if I took care of myself. Eventually, I'd have to start sticking myself with needles, and finally end up with so-called "deferred complications" anyway. This is known as the "natural course". All-natural, in other words. Anything else would be strange.

But are things really that bleak? Is there no alternative to facing the facts? Maybe there's hope to escape these problems, or at least delay them for a very long time?

I'm sure other diabetics have received the same brochures I did. What I didn't have, however, was a book that explained what had actually happened to me, and what problems I was about to face. The same book would obviously also tell me what to do to avoid the problems.

You're holding this "missing" book in your hands right now. This book is about what I wished I had known when I sat in the waiting room after my "sentence", waiting for my brochures and feeling confused. Yet, this book is meant not only for newly diagnosed and confused diabetics. Even if you have been living with diabetes for years and become accustomed to it, you will benefit from reading this book.

Improving your health will require some sacrifice, but most people will agree that it's worth it. After a while, many people no longer experience the sacrifice as something negative; on the contrary, they feel almost ashamed of it – it seems like a luxurious life. There are, of course, people who would rather take injections and eat their sandwiches; we have to accept this – even if it causes personal suffering and results in great expense to society.

The following pages will teach you enough to enable you to confidently reject advice that will only make you more ill.

The advice presented in this book is very different from what they write in the diabetes brochures. The advice in the brochures is based on the viewpoint that, of course, you should continue to eat more or less as you did before, just with more fibre and less fat. Almost all of the brochures are published by pharmaceutical companies, and they have no great desire to help you live without their medication. That's why their advice will slowly but surely make your condition worse, requiring more and more medication. As cynical as this may sound, it is the truth. This also applies to today's websites about diabetes. These are generally operated by pharmaceutical companies, and the advice presented there will keep you just sick enough to stay on your feet, but not to get well. I know this to be true.

Perhaps you remember the "Marlboro Man", Wayne Mc-Laren? The Marlboro Man was the cool cowboy featured in ads for Philip Morris' Marlboro cigarettes. McLaren smoked a pack and a half a day. He contracted lung cancer, and despite chemotherapy, radiation treatment and the removal of a lung, his life could not be saved. The cancer spread throughout his body and he died in July 1992. From his deathbed, he participated in an anti-smoking campaign, and the final phase of his suffering in the hospital was documented on film.

Wayne McLaren learned his lesson the hard way. Wilford Brimley was another man who paid a high price for his daily habits. Wilford was well-known in the United States for many television advertisements for Quaker Oats' Instant Oatmeal. In the TV ads, he portrayed a jolly old fellow who enjoyed spending time with his children and grandchildren, all the while praising the benefits of instant oatmeal. Maybe you can already guess what happened to him? Wilford Brimley contracted diabetes of course. These days, Wilford works for a supplier of diabetes treatment equipment.

It's not hard to imagine that at a relatively young age, you might promote something that's not good for you. You feel immortal. Wayne McLaren smoked cigarettes that destroyed his lungs and Wilford Brimley ate instant oatmeal.

Oatmeal contains starch, which is metabolised to glucose – the kind of sugar that elevates your blood sugar level. You might think that I'm saying that you can get diabetes from eating starch and sugar. It's really not quite that simple.

You cannot develop type 2 diabetes without eating sugar and starch. If you do eat sugar and starch, you can develop type 2 diabetes. But there's more to it than that. I'm convinced that a genetic predisposition is also necessary. In my case, one of my grandfathers had type 2 diabetes – I was genetically predisposed. However, if I hadn't gorged myself on potatoes and bread as I did, I'm sure that type 2 diabetes would not have developed. Instead, I would be walking around like a ticking diabetes bomb. That bomb would not have exploded, and so much the better for me. Instead, I was unlucky and developed type 2 diabetes.

If you avoid the disease-triggering factors, you won't get the disease. Just as a person who is predisposed to alcoholism can dodge the bullet by never drinking alcohol.

The advice presented in this book is based on the fact that you have decided to never suffer any symptoms of your diabetes, or at least reduce them as much you can.

The recommendations in the book focus mainly on what diabetics should eat to reduce their dependency on medication, so you will probably need to give up some of the foods you usually eat. It's your choice. You can follow the guidelines in the brochures you have received, increase your medication and still eat basically what you've always eaten. In time, as your weight increases, you will need to increase your medication – and in turn gain even more weight … and so on.

Some diabetes medications, such as sulfonylureas (also known as "SU" pills) and insulin make it harder to avoid gaining those extra pounds. When you start to eat according to the recommendations in this book, you're taking the most important step you can take to keep yourself healthy. I know of many cases where type 2 diabetes patients could stop taking medication and insulin after starting to eat the way I will describe in the following pages. Actually, there are also type 1 diabetics who can get by without insulin. As strange as it may sound, in some cases it's true.

As I previously implied, your new life may come to seem a bit luxurious, so if you're assuming that this new diet will be tedious and boring, you've got it all wrong. Instead, you'll be enjoying truly delicious meals.

In 1926, the Swedish journal *Hälsovännen (Friend of Health)* published a review of the book by Professor Karl Petrén entitled "On the Treatment of Diabetes (even with insulin)" by Georg Engstrand. Here are some quotes from the review:

"... few areas of medicine are in as dire need of a guide for treatment of the disease, as well as a general and accessible description of the disease's nature and essence, as is the case for diabetes. These patients must learn to understand their disease, and as it is to an exceptionally high degree influenced by the diet, it is similarly essential for the diabetic to understand the significance of the often rigorous regulations prescribed by the physician regarding the patient's diet.

Petrén's current presentation regarding the treatment of diabetics seems, in my opinion, to satisfactorily fulfil the requirements one may expect of such a document, both from the perspective of the physician and the patient. It must not be too superficial, but neither may it be scientifically complex, as it should be understood by a common labourer as well as satisfy the needs of the spiritually trained mind. In this regard, I consider Petren's work to be more than satisfactory, and I recommend it highly to anyone interested in this subject. In addition, Petren's work is useful as a guide to those physicians who are not specialised in this field."

It is my hope and desire that this book will function in a similar manner.

My story

The story of how I discovered THE SCANDINAVIAN DIET is truly frightening. THE SCANDINAVIAN DIET or LCHF (in Sweden) is short for Low-Carb, High-Fat. In other words, few carbohydrates and lots of fat. The thing is, after having grown as tall as I was going to get, my waistline continued to expand. I became quite husky, and as the years passed, I became quite thirsty as well. I loved to drink water, skimmed milk and orange juice.

I had come to the understanding that one could learn to drink plenty of fluids, and that drinking lots of water was good for your health. My thirst grew to bizarre proportions, but that's not why I sought help. The heel of my left foot had suddenly become more or less numb. My eyesight also began to deteriorate. It was during the examination of my heel that the doctors discovered I had type 2 diabetes – in other words, the "sugar disease".

I was immediately prescribed medication to reduce my blood sugar to an acceptable level. I was given Glucophage

(Metformin) as well as a second medication known as Mindiab. Glucophage causes the liver to secrete less sugar than it usually does; in addition, cells in the body become more sensitive to insulin, resulting in reduced insulin secretion. The reduced need for insulin makes it easier to keep your weight down, because insulin can cause weight gain. I've heard that Glucophage was originally intended to be used as a diet pill.

The other medication, Mindiab, causes the pancreas to release its insulin immediately. As a result, this medication can lower blood sugar levels very suddenly. One can feel clammy and shaky until one finds something sweet to eat. The high insulin levels also make it automatically harder to avoid gaining weight.

I actually noticed some serious symptoms the first morning I took Mindiab. A short while after I had swallowed the pill, my vision became blurred. I broke into a cold sweat and tremor, but I understood that it was probably due to low blood sugar, so I dragged myself to the refrigerator, grabbed a pitcher of orange juice and began to drink from it with great gulps. I lay down on the kitchen sofa and felt how the nasty sensation slowly disappeared.

I tried to follow the advice I was given. I ate very little fat, always choosing the leanest alternative. I have to admit that I didn't understand very much about diabetes at the time, nor did I think about it having anything to do with food. Professionals working with diabetes on a daily basis must know what they're doing, and I felt safe. Everything was so simple.

All of my meals were prepared according to the advice in the brochures, with just a few occasional lapses. I had oatmeal with half a grated apple each morning. I poured some skim milk over it and ate a whole-grain sandwich with low-fat margarine and a slice of low-fat cheese (which tasted like plastic). I was proud of my tasteless and boring diet in my certainty that I would be rewarded for it. Otherwise, what would be the point of being a good boy? In that case, I could just as well slurp down eggs and bacon for breakfast and never bother choosing the lean alternatives. For the first time in my life, I felt like a clean-living person, noting with some sense of superiority how others used full-fat spreads on their bread slices. Of course, I knew the importance of low-fat margarine.

My sense of well-being continued for about 10 months, when I suddenly suffered a heart attack. I knew that diabetics ran a higher risk of infarction than others, but I was still peeved because I had been eating such a healthy diet. I received a so-called stent implant in one of my coronary arteries. A coronary stent is a small stainless steel tube with slots. It props the artery open so that it cannot collapse and lead to another blockage.

This time, the coronary care nurse sternly told me that I needed to lose weight. Since my diabetes diagnosis almost a year previously, I had lost less than 5 pounds. To lose weight, I would have to eat even less fat than I had been.

This part seemed quite difficult. I wondered where I would find the fat that I would stop eating. As I was already choosing low-fat alternatives as a rule, this seemed virtually impossible. I concluded that all I could do was to stay on track and eat as little fat as I could.

About a year and a half later, still practising the low-fat

diet, I entered what is known as the "natural course of events". This is a process that diabetics go through – despite taking care of themselves. In practice this means that the blood sugar level goes up despite keeping to a strict and approved diet. More medication and, finally, insulin injections are required. Despite insulin injections, patients will experience the so-called deferred complications such as heart- and foot problems. We'll get back to these problems later.

I knew very little about how diabetes works, but I understood that it was serious. More and more often, my blood sugar reached high levels around lunchtime, despite two years on a low-fat diet. In other words, it was time to start taking medication to counter the high blood sugar, i.e. an SU (sulfonylurea) drug. These pills force the pancreas to secrete more insulin. That was when I started to seriously ponder how I would try to avoid my fate. I was told that I needed to lose weight in order to increase my insulin sensitivity. With better insulin sensitivity, I wouldn't need as much insulin to get the sugar in my blood to enter my muscle cells, where it could be of use and give me energy.

I needed to lose weight in order to improve my blood sugar levels and become healthier. Because I had consistently tried to avoid fat, I realised that avoiding fat was not the way to lose weight. Obviously, I needed to try something else. I began to search for information on the Internet about alternative ways to lose weight. After a while, I began to find sites that stated, for example, that it was not the white in the egg that was good for you, but rather the yolk! My first reaction, naturally, was that this must be a misprint, because I knew that the egg yolk was full of fat and cholesterol – in other words, a compressed clump of unhealthy stuff. The more I read, however, the more I began to realise that this was no misprint.

The documents I found recommended cutting down on carbohydrates and eating more natural fats instead. In some strange way, this would lead to shedding the pounds. That sounded crazy to me. It sounded so crazy that I decided to try it. The decision to start this seemingly backward diet was not easy. Eating full-fat butter and cream seemed less than logical. I mean, I was a heart patient already and had diabetes on top of that. All of the experts agreed that the diet I was about to adopt would be disastrous for a person like me. No sooner said than done. On September 15, 2003, I began to eat bacon and eggs for breakfast. For the rest of the day, I avoided carbohydrates. Before I had lost a single pound of fat, I experienced a dramatic improvement in my blood sugar levels. A few days later, I dared to stop taking the SU pills, and it turned out that I had better blood sugar levels when eating bacon and eggs without medication than when I ate oatmeal with skim milk and apple *with* medication!

Apparently, in my ignorance I had stumbled across something very valuable in ridding myself of diabetes symptoms. Without knowing it, I had started to eat food that did not raise my blood sugar levels. And that's the way it is. A lot of effort is being spent on discovering new medicines for diabetes treatment. Instead you can bring about the biggest changes on your own, simply by ignoring traditional dietary advice and doing the exact opposite. By skipping the oatmeal, potatoes, bread – even whole grain bread, pasta and rice, diabetics will notice a dramatic improvement. Many people have been able to stop taking their medication; sometimes completely. In any case, anyone can reduce their medication by switching from the recommended diet to THE SCANDINAVIAN DIET.

What is diabetes?

To develop a good understanding, we should first look at what diabetes actually is. You probably know that diabetes is related to a disturbance in blood sugar levels. A healthy person can eat a doughnut, and the blood sugar level will decrease rapidly afterwards; for a diabetic, however, this takes a long time. High blood sugar levels will harm the body. We'll delve deeper into that later.

There are several types of diabetes. You have probably heard of type 1- and type 2 diabetes. There is also pregnancy-related diabetes and an intermediate form that initially resembles type 2 diabetes, but after some years becomes type 1 diabetes. This type is called LADA. However, type 2 diabetes is by far the most common.

The medical term is *diabetes mellitus*. The word "diabetes" loosely means "to pass through", and the word "mellitus" means "honey". Diabetes mellitus loosely means that the patient drinks a lot and produces a lot of urine, which is sweet. Not so long ago, doctors would taste the urine to determine if a patient had diabetes! This method of diagnosis has, thankfully, been abandoned.

So, the elevated sugar level in the blood causes the diabetic's problems. In order to reduce the blood sugar level, the body needs *insulin*. Insulin is produced by the pancreas and is released into the body when blood sugar levels are high. Insulin causes the cells of the body to absorb sugar from the blood, resulting in reduced blood sugar levels.

Insulin is the only hormone in the body that can reduce blood sugar levels. The name "insulin" comes from the Latin word for "island". Actually, the part of the pancreas called the *Islets of Langerhans* is responsible for the production of insulin. There, the insulin producing cells, which are also the most numerous, are known as *beta cells*. There are also *alpha cells*, which produce another hormone called *glucagon*. Glucagon acts to increase blood sugar levels. The blood sugar level determines how much insulin (which acts to lower the blood sugar level) is released. In turn, insulin regulates the release of glucagon.

Let's take a closer look at the most common forms of diabetes.

Type 1

In type 1 diabetes, the disease presents itself in the form of dangerously high blood sugar levels as a result of insufficient insulin production. In other words, there's not enough insulin to suppress the level of blood sugar.

Type 1 diabetes is a so-called autoimmune disease. This autoimmune disease causes the body to suddenly perceive its own insulin-producing beta cells as intruders, and literally attacks them. With no insulin, the blood sugar level becomes dangerously high.

Many type 1 diabetics have some residual production of new insulin-producing beta cells, but these are continually destroyed by the autoimmune disease. The end result is that there are always a few beta cells producing insulin while they wait to be destroyed. When those cells are gone, new beta cells are produced. In other words, a few functioning beta cells can help a type 1 diabetic get by on a minimum of insulin, without injections. Of course, eating right is also necessary.

Strangely enough, low blood sugar can also occur in the diabetic. When a diabetic takes an insulin injection to lower the blood sugar level, the amount of insulin can sometimes be more than necessary for the amount of consumed carbohydrates and proteins. Virtually all type 1 diabetics need insulin injections, but even type 2 diabetics with dysfunctional insulin production may need to inject insulin. If too much insulin is injected, blood sugar levels may decrease so much that the diabetic falls into a coma. Even high blood sugar levels can lead to coma, but the most common cause of coma in diabetics is low blood sugar.

As a matter of fact, airline flight attendants are instructed to assume that a diabetic passenger who has lapsed into a coma is suffering from low blood sugar, and they should take appropriate action themselves (if there is no doctor on board). They are taught to administer something sweet to bring the blood sugar up to a reasonable level. To counter a low blood sugar situation, one should administer the equivalent of three glucose tablets. This is equivalent to about 200ml (7 fl oz) milk or 100ml (3.5 fl oz) juice. As you can see, both milk and juice contain relatively large amounts of sugar, and if one is to keep one's blood sugar levels within a safe range, both of these should be consumed with considerable care.

Type 2

Type 2-diabetes should in reality be called by its original name – "the sugar disease". It really is the sugar that causes the diabetic's problems. For type 2 diabetics who do not inject insulin or take sulfonylureas, the problem is virtually always high blood sugar levels. Sulfonylureas are often referred to as SU-preparations or SU pills because "sulfonylureas" can be somewhat difficult to pronounce. This medication squeezes insulin from the pancreas on demand. That's why it's extremely rare that a type 2 diabetic *without* SU pills or insulin injections lapses into a coma due to low blood sugar levels.

The type 2 diabetic usually has normal or even elevated insulin production, but this does not help when the muscle cells do not react to the insulin. Sugar stays in the blood and causes trouble. The specific insulin receptors on the cells have stopped reacting.

The type 2 diabetic's cells become less and less sensitive to insulin over time. As a result, a diabetic will release huge amounts of insulin to try to force the cells to react.

**High insulin levels promote fat storage
and slow down the utilization of stored fat.**

The effect of insulin is to reduce fat metabolism while simultaneously promoting fat storage. Because muscle cells become insulin-resistant while fat cells do not (to any significant degree), sugar is absorbed into fat cells for a lack of anywhere else to go. The result is that these fat cells get bigger. That's why diabetics are often obese.

There are, however, type 2 diabetics who are thin. Thin type 2 diabetics (about 20%) may suffer from type 1-like diabetes; they produce the antibodies that attack beta cells, but their insulin production is nevertheless sufficient to manage without additional insulin. The insulin level that promotes fat storage is low, and that's why they don't gain weight. The thinner a person is, the higher their sensitivity to insulin. Because thin type 2 diabetics do not become overweight, the small amount of insulin that is nevertheless present may still be enough to help lower blood sugar levels.

LADA
(Latent Autoimmune Diabetes of Adults)

LADA is a slowly progressing form of type 1 diabetes. In its early stages, LADA appears to be a type 2 diabetes, but as the disease progresses, insulin production ceases just as it does in type 1 diabetes.

Summary

Insulin lowers blood sugar by signalling the body's cells to absorb glucose from the bloodstream. Insulin also inhibits fat metabolism and promotes fat storage in the body.

Type 1 diabetes is caused by the body's inability to produce the insulin that reduces blood sugar levels. When blood sugar cannot enter the cells, it stays in the bloodstream, and sugar levels become high enough to cause injury.

Type 2 diabetes is caused by the body's muscle cells not being able to react to insulin, thus leaving sugar to circulate in the bloodstream.

LADA is a form of diabetes that initially appears to be type 2, but after a number of years LADA progresses to type 1 diabetes because insulin production is insufficient or stops completely.

Complications

Now I'm going to talk about deferred complications. What happens to blood vessels, nerves, kidneys, eyes and coronary vessels etc. when blood sugar levels are not under control?

This is not a pleasant section – basically miserable. Well, let's be done with it. Let's have a look at the problems diabetes can cause. Too much sugar in your blood is not that dangerous when it's just for a short time. It's when blood sugar is elevated for a prolonged time that the body can suffer serious injury in various ways. One can usually notice high blood sugar levels by a dry mouth, thirst and a frequent need to urinate. Some people experience fatigue. Sometimes one notices impaired vision or numbness.

Inflammation

High blood sugar in combination with high insulin levels causes inflammation in the body. What, then, is *inflammation*? The word inflammation comes from the Latin word for fire, which helps explain what's happening. If a wound becomes inflamed, it hurts. Blood flow to the area is increased, causing redness and elevated temperature. Inflammation is the body's way of protecting itself against invaders. Inflammation is painful because fluid from the blood enters the tissue around the area and causes it to tighten. Inflammation in blood vessel walls dramatically increases the risk for coronary disease. You might have heard that people with diabetes have a higher risk for coronary diseases such as heart attacks and strokes. It's this tendency to increased inflammation in the blood vessels that causes the increased risk.

Not only blood vessels are affected; nerves can also become inflamed. When a skin wound is inflamed, you know that it's healing, and after a while you can't even tell that there was an injury there. Unfortunately, inflamed nerves do not always heal equally well. They don't "regenerate". For example, damaged nerves in the feet may not heal completely. Because the tiny blood vessels in the feet can be seriously injured, it's not altogether uncommon that amputation is necessary to save the rest of the body.

Eyes

The microvessels in the retina are in danger of injury from diabetes. High blood sugar damages the vessels in the retina, making it extremely important to keep blood sugar levels at a safe level. The resulting injury can include impaired vision or blindness. During a 15 year period, about 10% of diabetes patients will experience visual impairment. I hope we can change that now. Still, many diabetics have lived significantly longer with their disease without suffering from any visual impairment. Injury to the retina occurs before the diabetic even notices it. That's why it's important for a diabetic to not waste any time getting an eye exam.

It's normal for a diabetes patient to have regular eye exams in order to discover any changes. This is generally done by retinal photography. The retinal photograph is then compared to previously taken images, which will reveal any signs of injury that should be addressed.

One could say that the fine vessels develop aneurysms; there are bulges in the blood vessel walls. These bulges cause the vessels to become more fragile, possibly resulting in blood leakage into the retina. This can in turn cause the retina to swell and bleed, also entailing a risk of blockage in the vessels. Swelling is noticeable in the form of blurred and/or distorted vision. If a blood vessel is occluded (blocked) near the macula, (oval-shaped yellow spot near the centre of the retina), the injury may lead to vision loss. Such injuries may often heal on their own, provided that blood sugar is kept at a low and constant level.

If the tiny vessels are repeatedly blocked, the retina can experience something similar to an infarction or obstructed blood vessel. This results in oxygen deprivation to the retina. As in the heart, new blood vessels can form to assist the injured and insufficient old vessels, but the new vessels are not as efficient as the originals, sort of like an inferior quality knockoff. They tend to leak blood, which can even lead to retinal detachment.

Kidneys

Kidney injury linked to diabetes is called *nephrotic syndrome*. Just as with eye injury, some patients seem to avoid it whereas others do not.

Although the kidneys participate in blood formation, their best-known function is to clear the body of toxins and other metabolic by-products. About 400 gallons of blood pass through the kidneys every day! In addition, the kidneys regulate blood pressure and monitor the fluid-, pH- and calcium balance. This balance is referred to as *homeostasis*. The body constantly strives to be in balance. If you start to feel chilly, your brain will start to nag you to put on more clothing. If your body is dehydrated, you'll feel thirsty and forget everything else until you get a drink of water. These examples represent things that you can control yourself, but many regulatory systems in the body maintain balance without you thinking about them or even being able to consciously affect them. Kidney functions are an example of the latter.

The kidneys contain masses of tangles of tiny blood vessels, or capillaries. When everything works as it should, these capillaries filter the blood, removing waste products from the body via the urine. They can do this because the capillaries are partially permeable, which means that fluids and salts can pass through their walls. When these tangles of capillaries – or *glomeruli* as they are known – are injured due to excessively high blood sugar for a prolonged time, the capillary walls are damaged. They basically develop holes. This in turn leads to

37

small amounts of proteins escaping through the holes in the capillary walls. When blood proteins can reach the urine in this way, it is referred to as microalbuminuria. Protein in the urine is not in itself harmful, but it is a sign of kidney damage.

In the long run, kidney damage can require dialysis, which means that the blood must be purified in a special apparatus. Kidney transplants are another solution. Both the kidney and the pancreas can be transplanted at the same time. In this way, the patient will not need to take insulin. Surgery, however, is always risky. A pancreas transplant is especially tricky.

Most kidney damage is probably caused by high insulin levels in combination with insulin resistance. This is often the result of prolonged high blood sugar levels. High protein intake has no significance for kidney damage. Eating too much protein is still not wise, because excess dietary protein is converted to glucose and will elevate blood sugar levels. If kidney damage is serious, it can also contribute to high levels of hazardous nitrogen metabolites in the blood.

Teeth

As a diabetic, your risk of dental problems is twice that of others. A diabetic's mouth is more prone to infection. Infections can also promote coronary disease.

One factor required for loosening of the teeth – periodontitis – is plaque. Plaque is a bacterial film that forms on the teeth and the edges of the gums. Plaque that is not removed can harden and form tartar. Tartar is somewhat porous and can in turn provide fertile ground for continued bacterial growth. Excessive bacteria in the mouth can lead to inflammation between the teeth and gums. When this kind of inflammation occurs in the gums, white blood cells – leukocytes – are mobilised to stop the infection. However, the white blood cells in diabetics do not work as efficiently as in healthy people. For this reason, diabetics are more prone to inflammation than others. Like salt on a wound, a negative spiral begins when the infection itself raises blood sugar levels. The body goes on red alert when it must deal with an infection, which means that blood sugar-elevating hormones such as adrenaline and cortisol are released. The increased blood sugar provides the body with the energy it needs to battle the infection.

Elevated blood sugar damages the tiny blood vessels in the mouth and ultimately causes teeth to loosen. The elevated blood sugar reduces oxygen supply to the tissue, increasing the risk of periodontitis.

When the mouth becomes inflamed, the tissues secrete fluid with a high sugar concentration, as sugar levels in the blood of diabetics are generally higher. This can also lead to cavities. The saliva itself can also be sweet in a diabetic, further increasing the risk. High sugar concentration in the saliva can also result in *thrush*, an oral fungal infection. This can cause pain, sores and deposits. Just as with other fungal infections, sugar promotes thrush infections.

Coronary disease

Diabetics are more prone to coronary disease than most others. About half of all diabetic patients die prematurely from heart disease. Half, or almost half, of non-diabetics also die of heart disease. This can come in the form of angina pectoris, which is experienced as chest pains. This occurs most often after vigorous exercise. A more serious variant is a heart attack. A heart attack occurs when a coronary blood vessel is blocked enough to prevent blood from supplying the heart with oxygen. As a result, part of the heart muscle can "die". The heart may continue to beat, but is not as strong. Serious heart attacks can be fatal – sudden cardiac death.

Heart attacks – how they work

The most reasonable explanation I have heard regarding how and why people develop atherosclerosis and suffer subsequent heart attacks was presented by Uffe Ravnskov.

As previously mentioned, a heart attack occurs when a blood vessel in the heart becomes sufficiently obstructed to prevent blood from passing through. The obstruction is actually not caused by the hardening of the arteries, but rather when a small bubble in the blood vessel wall (called a "vulnerable plaque"), bursts. According to Ravnskov, these bubbles in blood vessel walls (which we have known about for many years) are actually boils.

In reality, we continually inhale viruses and bacteria; we

eat them in our food and they can gain entry via our eyes or through wounds. These foreign microbes – viruses and bacteria – constitute the actual basis of a heart attack, or infarct. They only appear in the arteries.

After the microbes have entered the body, they are attacked by the body's defences; our immune system. The immune system consists of several parts, one of which is the type of white blood cells known as macrophages.

Invaders are promptly killed by white blood cells after being neutralised by our antibodies. Another method, which few of us know about, is immobilization with the help of lipoproteins. When an invader shows up in the body, a signal is sent to the liver to create more lipoproteins – these are the carriers of cholesterol. Synthesis of lipoproteins also includes those known as LDLs. Maybe you've heard about cholesterol, and that HDL is healthy and LDL is not. It's quite a mystery how they came up with the idea that LDLs are harmful to your body when they are produced by the liver. It's as if a country would train a hostile army with the express purpose of attacking its own territory...

In any case, lipoproteins are an effective defence mechanism. LDL-cholesterol sacrifices itself by adhering to the invading microbe. LDL-cholesterol molecules that have caught an invader stick together and create clumps. They can sometimes become too large to pass through the finely meshed network of capillaries that supply arterial walls with oxygen and nutrients, because the pressure outside the walls of the arterial capillaries is quite high. In the capillaries surrounding veins, the clumps pass through much more easily because the pressure is lower. This is probably one of the reasons that there is no hardening of veins, only of arteries.

Well, enough of that. After LDL molecules have captured a microbe, they clump together with other LDLs that have done the same. In the next step, a white blood cell, or macrophage, rushes in to "swallow" the LDL/microbe clumps. Apparently, macrophages think that LDLs with microbes stuck on them look strange, and need to be swallowed. Macrophages can distinguish between regular LDL-cholesterols and those that have taken "prisoners". It seems that macrophages don't devour lone LDL molecules out on patrol. That is, unless the macrophages feel that they need more cholesterol; then the lone LDLs can be threatened.

After having been captured, special enzymes will chop the microbe/LDL aggregates into small pieces. If poisonous or foreign particles are present, the macrophages also call for additional flow of blood and lymph. When this happens, we experience what is known as inflammation. Inflammation can be necessary for the body to successfully defend itself against harmful invaders. When a macrophage engulfs the cell, it's known as *phagocytosis*. When cholesterol from the LDL has been digested in the macrophage, it's recycled to create new cholesterol, which is transported to the liver by HDL.

This is what happens when everything works as it should. The body defeats the invaders. This is not particularly dramatic, it's going on all the time in your body while you're reading this, and is completely normal.

So, how can things go wrong? Well, if the immune system is suppressed, macrophages are not able to do their jobs. Then the invading microbes gain the upper hand. If the capillaries in the arterial walls are completely blocked by clumps of LDL, a piece of the arterial wall dies. Microbes can then enter the arterial tissue, multiply and convert the piece of dead tissue into a microscopic boil – a vulnerable plaque. In other words, dead arterial wall sections together with microbes turn into boils.

When one of these boils bursts, its contents of microbes, cholesterol and other stuff enters the artery and travels in to the heart muscle; a blood clot is also created on the edge of the newly ruptured plaque. This blood clot first causes pain, which is followed by injury to the heart muscle. The worst-case scenario after an infarct is death, when the heart doesn't receive enough oxygen to do its job.

Stent

Another risk factor to be considered is the mesh tube that is often implanted in the constricted blood vessel. These are called stents and are often made of stainless steel. At the age of 43, after sticking to the diet recommended for diabetics, I suffered a heart attack. Two blood vessels had been obstructed. They were both dilated using balloon angioplasty, and the stent was implanted in one of them to prevent it from another blockage.

The stents can, however, present a real danger. They are supposed to reduce the risk of new infarcts; unfortunately, it's not that simple. Seven years later, I began to experience recurring pain in my heart, enough to convince me to seek medical treatment. An examination revealed that, of the two obstructed blood vessels, that been the one that had been treated with balloon angioplasty was fine, whereas the vessel that had received the stent implant was once again constricted. The medical term for this is *restenosis*.

It's not unusual for stainless steel stents to cause these problems. Alas, yet another area of medicine that needs more attention. This treatment method continues to be used with no particular regard for the results.

The Lancet (2000, pp 1895–1897) published a study about stents and the possible results of their use. In this study, a number of patients with stent implants were re-examined six months after surgery. Of the patients who displayed allergic reactions to nickel, molybdenum and chrome, 100% had experienced symptoms so severe that they required additional surgery at the site of the implant. Of those who did not display allergic symptoms, 57% required additional treatment for constriction in the stent. Not only is the stent a risk factor, it is by far the greatest risk factor in this scenario.

Now, I have learned to take Trombyl (a blood coagulation inhibitor), which I had not taken for years. I was feeling fine, and had no idea that the stent itself could be dangerous to my health.

In any case, seven years had passed without any problems. Aside from the stent, the rest of the blood vessels in my heart looked fine. It was the foreign object that caused the problem. All I need to do now is to continue eating natural foods in order to delay any problems, in addition to taking my Trombyl. I don't think the stent can be just simply removed. So, my advice to those of you who have had this piece of metal implanted is to use Trombyl to reduce the risk of future problems.

Gastroparesis

People with diabetes are prone to nerve injury. This can cause a number of problems. In our bodies we have something called the "autonomous nervous system". These nerves control those bodily functions that are not under conscious control. For example, our heart and liver. They also control gastro-intestinal functions, and make the intestines move around to shift the food downwards towards the exit.

Diabetes can injure nerves – even those in the stomach. Because of this, the stomach may not be able to mix and churn food as well as it should. This will lead to food be-ing transported out of the stomach too slowly. The narrow outlet of the stomach (pylorum) becomes more or less para-lysed, a condition known as *gastroparesis*. Nerve damage from diabetes can also lead to loss of sensation in the lower intestine and sphincter, making it difficult to control the bowels.

Gastroparesis has various symptoms which can appear and disappear. Sometimes it's diarrhoea, sometimes it's con-stipation. Stomach pains might appear directly after a meal or maybe late at night. In healthy persons, the narrow outlet of the stomach opens more during the night to allow larger food chunks to continue through the digestive system; gastro-paresis prevents this nocturnal opening of the valve. With gastroparesis, food accumulates in the stomach, causing problems.

Digestion is also affected by blood sugar levels. The stomach empties at a slower rate when blood sugar is high and at a faster rate when blood sugar is low. Because diabetics often have high blood sugar levels, stomach emptying will be slower.

Gastroparesis can cause the sensation that the stomach is full, despite having eaten very little. You might feel nauseous and want to vomit after eating.

Sexual impairment

Both women and men can experience sexual problems due to diabetes. Man can suffer from impotence, whereas women can experience vaginal dryness, making sexual intercourse painful. These problems may be due to a malfunction in nerve signalling. Nerve damage is a very serious problem in diabetes.

Foot problems

Problems with the feet are a very common complication in diabetes. There can be several reasons for this. For example, nerves in the feet can be damaged. One sign of this is numbness in the feet. Other foot injuries can go unnoticed for a long time, resulting in slow-healing infections.

Problems can also be due to poor blood circulation in the feet. Blood vessels can, as we know, be damaged by elevated blood sugar. If this happens, the feet will not get the oxygen they need, and sores on the feet will heal slowly or not at all. For oxygen to reach the tissue, nitric oxide must act on the blood vessels to dilate them. High blood sugar leads to poor distribution of nitric oxide, resulting in constricted blood vessels and less oxygen reaching the tissues.

Infections also cause foot injuries, mostly due to the fact that diabetics are more sensitive to infections than others. If there are deformities on the feet, these can also promote injury; for example, blisters, calluses or simple sores, which also are more prone to serious infection.

Serious problems may require amputation. It is sometimes not enough to remove one or several toes; in serious cases, the entire foot or lower leg is amputated.

Frozen shoulder

A condition known as frozen shoulder is not uncommon in diabetics, even if others can also suffer from it. It usually appears between the ages of 40 and 60, and is characterised by pain in one shoulder. The pain is initially severe, but gradually becomes more like a grinding and nagging pain, accompanied by reduced mobility in the shoulder. The pain and stiffness can persist for several years before disappearing.

The cause of frozen shoulder is unknown. It is, however, an inflammatory disease that attacks the shoulder capsule and also affects the surrounding muscles.

Alzheimer's

Diabetics have a greater risk than others of developing Alzheimer's disease, a severe form of dementia. The cause of Alzheimer's disease is not known, but there are several theories regarding potential causes of this disease. It is known that prior to the disease, a substance known as beta amyloid is formed around nerve cells in the brain. Beta amyloid should normally be cleaned out by a "housekeeper" called IDE. The housekeeper's primary task is to remove insulin, and in individuals with high insulin levels, the housekeeper may not be capable of cleaning up both the beta amyloids and the insulin, as a result of which the beta amyloids remain in place and in time lead to the development of Alzheimer's disease. Medical researchers in the field have referred to Alzheimer's disease as type 3 diabetes. This is still a theory which has not yet been proven.

How is diabetes described?

According to the diabetes brochure, a type 2 diabetic can expect to experience the "natural course of events". In other words, the diabetic can initially eat a sugar- and white bread-free diet, and later start to take Metformin. This medication is said to increase the sensitivity of the cells to insulin. It also prevents sugar from being secreted from the liver too easily. Every morning, the liver secretes sugar (among other things); we probably evolved this way to have the energy to chase down fresh mammoth for breakfast. This sugar dose is bad news for the diabetic, who has a hard time managing the elevated blood sugar level.

After Metformin is no longer sufficient, the next step is to start taking one of the SU preparations, which causes the pancreas to secrete more insulin. This helps transport sugar from the blood into the cells. One problem with switching to medication that increases insulin secretion is that it can cause sudden drops in blood sugar levels. The body's own regulatory mechanisms are bypassed, and an insulin dose is generated by force. As you recall, insulin also inhibits fat metabolism, thus promoting fat storage. So, when the extra insulin secretion begins, type 2 diabetics will have a really hard time keeping their body weight down. Increased weight means reduced insulin sensitivity, requiring even more insulin to get the body to react.

The next step is to start to inject insulin. This happens when the pancreas cannot create enough insulin, not even when it's being stimulated by the SU pills.

Type 2 diabetics with no history of overweight will testify to the fact that when insulin injections start, gaining weight really becomes a problem; this is related to insulin's effect on fat metabolism.

Diabetes brochures generally tell us which foods are good for a diabetic. Diabetics are encouraged to eat a low-fat, high-fiber diet, and to eat only the so-called "slow carbs". Because the diabetic should still eat carbs (!), even if carbs are exactly the problem. Slow carbs will let you live longer, because blood sugar levels rise slower than with fast carbs. It seems that none of the brochure authors have hit upon the idea that you should simply avoid the food that makes you sick.

They usually also tell you what happens if one doesn't succeed in keeping blood sugar levels under control. However, failure to control blood sugar levels is actually caused by following the very same advice from the brochure. Keeping blood sugar levels under control requires the courage to stand up against the advice about slow carbs.

When attempts to control the blood sugar level have completely failed, the so-called *deferred complications* begin, which I referred to previously in this book.

I found a link to a film about diabetes on the Swedish Diabetes Association's homepage. A professor was informing us about the two most common types of diabetes. Among other things, she tells us that it usually takes 10 to 15 years before a patient needs to begin injecting insulin. She explains why people get type 2 diabetes; that it's mostly due to genetic factors. Weight gain, smoking, stress, not enough sleep and exercise also increase the risk for diabetes. It seems that the professor does not believe that diet has any noteworthy effect.

We then see footage of a man who has had diabetes since the early 1990s. Although he takes insulin, he says that there is hope because new medicines are being developed all the time. There is still no mention of which foods might help control blood sugar levels. As the film goes on, the narrator shifts the focus to medication.

According to the introductory credits, it is a collaborative effort between the Swedish Diabetes Association and Adaption Media. Another producer of the film is www.netdoktor.se, a Swedish health web site. Netdoktor.se has this past year been sponsored by and featured advertisements for:

Aco Hud, Abbott, AFA, Allt om linser, Apoteket, Astma & Allergiförbundet, Astra Zeneca Sverige, Bayer, Biomade, Boehringer Ingelham, Braun, Bristol-Myers Squibb, Cancerfonden, Cederroth, Eli Lilly, Folksam, Försäkringskassan, Glaxo, H Lundbeck, Janssen-Cilag, Kellogg´s, Merck Sharp & Dohme, Motvärk, Nodensa, Novartis, Novo Nordisk, Nycomed, Organon, Procter & Gamble, Pfizer, Recip, Roche, Röda korset, Sanofi-Aventis, Sanofi Pasteur MSD, SCA Hygiene Products, SOS-barnbyar, Unipath, Unicef, Vitalas, Wyeth and Årstiderna.

This list includes quite a motley crew of drug manufacturers, who, naturally, are mainly interested in selling as much of their product as possible for as long as possible. Embarrassingly enough, Kellogg's is also among them. Kellogg's' products are outstanding when it comes to raising blood sugar levels, creating problems for anyone who has difficulty keeping blood sugar levels on an even keel. Novo Nordisk, who profits from selling insulin and injection equipment, is another sponsor.

One might ask if there are any non-profit motives for their sponsorship. Do they want patients to regain their health and not need their medicine? What image are they trying to project? Do they actually want patients to stop having to test their blood sugar all the time? Why is there no mention in the film about food, diet and health? Why do they instead talk about medication while panning and zooming through images of various delicious baked goods? Can it really be true that nobody involved in making the film believes that blood sugar levels and diabetes are affected by what you eat?

You don't need to be a rocket scientist to realise that pharmaceutical companies need to make a profit, even if that means keeping the public in the dark about certain types of diabetes treatment. What really irks me, however, is that they still pretend to be the "good guys", out to do us a good turn. Of course they don't want us to get well, but it would be even worse for business if they didn't pretend to care about us. What it really boils down to is exploitation of sick people, cashing in on them for as long as possible. I guess this is just business as usual for a pharmaceutical company. But still, I think they should lay their cards on the table.

Society would benefit immensely if more people realised what their game was. More people would be willing to try other ways to get a grip on their diabetes problems.

Wise old Buddha told us that "Wisdom shouldn't be simply respected, it needs to be put to the test." While reading this book, you shouldn't simply believe everything I say; on the contrary, I hope you will be inspired to ask more questions. Don't forget who is making money on the drugs you take.

What is a diabetic expected to do?

The diabetic is naturally expected to follow the dietary advice he or she is given. This means that the lion's share of their daily energy will be supplied by carbohydrates. The reason the diabetic should consume what he or she does not tolerate is to avoid eating too much fat.

We have been taught to believe that too much fat will result in high cholesterol, which in turn will cause a heart attack. This two-stage rocket takes us to the conclusion that fat – especially saturated fat – is bad for us. No such direct link has ever been demonstrated. Most of the evidence actually points to natural animal fats being beneficial to the cardiovascular system. The fat-eating Inuits do not suffer from heart disease when following their traditional diet. Considering the huge amount of fat they eat, one might naturally assume that they would be plagued with heart disease.

Nor do people generally think that a high blood sugar level is a problem that should be tackled head-on. The problem should disappear gradually by reducing carbohydrates in the diet. Like beating around the bush, insulin sensitivity would improve by reducing the patient's weight. Getting rid of a pot belly would lead to better sensitivity to insulin. And "everybody" knows that one can't lose weight by eating fat. And if one cannot eat fat, one must eat *something else*. This *something else* will, I presume, contain carbohydrates. Of the available nutrients, carbohydrates are most efficient at making a diabetic sicker. In addition, losing weight becomes more difficult, which, oddly enough, was the whole idea of not eating fat.

According to this, the astronomical blood sugar levels caused by the carbohydrate diet would then be countered by insulin injections and – hey presto! – the problem is solved! In other words, have as many jelly beans as you want. A fistful of jelly beans in one hand and a syringe in the other.

The diabetic's problems will now include both high sugar levels and high insulin levels. A good comparison would be to drive a car while flooring the gas and stomping hard on the brake at the same time. This sounds crazy, and it sure is. It is just as crazy as eating sugar and starch, which elevates blood sugar levels to a maximum (flooring it), and then injecting insulin (stomping on the brake) to get a good average "speed".

I'll show you that, by not pressing the accelerator as much, one need not brake as much either. Your body will feel better and thank you by letting you feel better. As an additional bonus, you won't need the insulin (that promotes fat storage), which will help you keep your weight down.

Science of Nutrition

Before we can know what diabetics should really eat, we need to know the basics about the so-called macronutrients: carbohydrates, fat and protein. The body uses fat and protein to make glucose, among other things. Glucose is essential for our bodies. Some people insist that we need to eat carbohydrates (which contain glucose) so that our brains can function. This is wrong; we can create our own glucose. This means that we don't need carbohydrates for a fulfilled, complete life. We only need to eat proteins and fat.

Fat

Imagine a section of a string of beads. Let it represent a string of carbon atoms bound to each other. The string of beads can be of various lengths. There is a hydrogen atom sitting on either side of each carbon atom. In simple terms, this is what a saturated fatty acid looks like. Because it's saturated, each carbon atom has two hydrogen atoms attached to it. In other words, there are no free spaces. This makes the fat molecule quite rigid at room temperature – if the fatty acids are short.

There are plenty of saturated fats in food from animals. Coconut is the only fruit that contains high levels of saturated fat.

Then we have the unsaturated fats. In monounsaturated fats, there is a double bond between two carbons, resulting in two fewer hydrogen atoms. Because the carbon chain is not fully loaded with hydrogen atoms, the fatty acid is "bent" and cannot be packed together with other chains as effectively as the saturated fats. This can be seen by its higher viscosity; monounsaturated fat is liquid at room temperature.

Polyunsaturated fats, however, have double bonds and fewer hydrogen atoms in two or more places.

Some types of unsaturated fats have special functions. For example, we have the omega-3 fats, which have an anti-inflammatory action. We call them omega-3 fats because there is a double bond between the third and fourth carbon atom, counting from the far end. "Omega" is the physiologist's name for the end from which we begin counting. If the double bond is after the sixth carbon atom from the omega end, the fat is referred to as omega-6. Omega-3 and omega-6 interact with each other. It is thought that there should be a proper balance between omega-3 and omega-6.

You'd imagine that it might be better with even more omega-3, so we would be less susceptible to inflammation? Actually, when the body is attacked, inflammation is often necessary to fight off the attackers. Too much omega-3 can suppress the protective inflammatory mechanism. In reality, the food we regularly stuff into our mouths has up to 15 – 20 times more omega-6 fat than we actually need. In other words, we eat food that promotes internal inflammation.

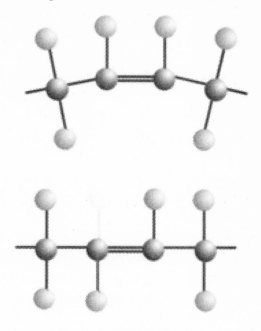

Cis- and trans-fats

Trans-fats are a specific type of fat. If you imagine a fatty acid where the two hydrogen atoms beside the double bond are next to each other, this is called the *cis-form*. If you instead move the hydrogen atom over from the one side to the other, you would have the trans-form. *Trans* means "on the other side" or "to the other side", telling us how the hydrogen atoms are oriented. This enables the fatty acid to retain its straight form and thus be solid at room temperature. This transformation can be done in the laboratory, producing an artificial trans-fatty acid. There are also natural trans-fats in products from ruminants such as cattle. Cream can contain trans-fat. Still, there is a difference between natural and artificial trans-fats. According to professor Göran Petersson at the Chalmers Institute, natural trans-fats are known to help protect against various forms of cancer and atherosclerosis (hardening of the arteries).

When polyunsaturated fat is hardened, the omega-3 form is the first to disappear. Omega-3 is in the type of fat most people need more of to counterbalance the large intake of omega-6.

Swedish health authorities generally group trans-fats together with saturated fats, even though they are very different by definition. It's like comparing apples and billiard balls. There is a scientifically unfounded opinion that we should minimise our intake of both saturated fat and trans-fat. That's why they're lumped in the same group.

Nor is there any discrimination between natural and artificial trans-fats. There seems to be no end to the number of ways the general public is fooled into eating, let's say, low-fat margarine.

In Sweden today, store-bought margarine does not contain trans-fat. Industrial margarine, on the other hand, may still contain trans-fat. Store-bought crackers, cakes and cookies regularly contain trans-fat. Products containing trans-fat have a much longer shelf life. That's why you can buy a box of cookies and they'll keep fresh for 10 years. In contrast to the Danish authorities, the Swedish authorities have not deemed it necessary to pass legislation limiting trans-fats. In Sweden, the food industry makes these decisions.

Protein

Proteins serve many different functions in the body. These include transport, structural and cell-repair functions. Proteins are made up of amino acids; in humans, there are 20 different types of amino acids. A bit less than half of them are essential amino acids, meaning that we cannot make them ourselves, and they must therefore be present in our food. Proteins that contain all the essential amino acids are known as "complete" proteins. Complete proteins can only be found in animal products such as meat, fish, eggs, cheese and the like. They aren't present in vegetable-based foods such as soy burgers. That is why animal-based foods are highly recommended.

If there is too much protein in the diet, the excess is converted to glucose – blood sugar. What does that mean? Well, it means that your blood sugar levels goes up. And when the blood sugar level goes up, extra insulin is secreted to get it down again. For a diabetic, this will promote weight gain, and for a type 2 diabetic, increased insulin resistance. Then, even more of the fat-storing insulin is secreted. That's why we should be careful not to eat more protein than we need.

Carbohydrates

Carbohydrates can be divided into three types: sugar, starch (sugar chains) and dietary fibre. We don't need to eat any of these (see page 64).

Sugar

The type of sugar that elevates blood sugar is called glucose. If you eat a sugar cube, you will be swallowing sucrose (also known as saccharose). Sucrose is made up of one molecule of glucose and one molecule of fructose. This means that when you eat a sugar cube, not all of the sugar in it will raise your blood sugar level. Only the half that is glucose. The rest, the fructose, goes directly to the liver and is stored as reserve fuel, called glycogen. When the liver is already filled with glycogen, it converts fructose to fat. Fat is stored in the liver and in other places in the body.

When geese are force-fed corn to produce *pâté de foie gras*, a fatty liver is induced. Some people consider this a delicacy. The carbohydrates are responsible for the fatty liver.

Maybe you've heard that fructose is especially fattening? The reason for this is that the liver transforms fructose into fat. Fruits contain about equal amounts of fructose and glucose, so that the fruit basket that generous employers might provide is not as good for their employees' fitness as one might think. If a type 2 diabetic eats plenty of fruit, the glucose will cause a blood sugar surge and the fructose will cause weight

RECOMMENDED DAILY ALLOWANCE

www.dietdoctor.com

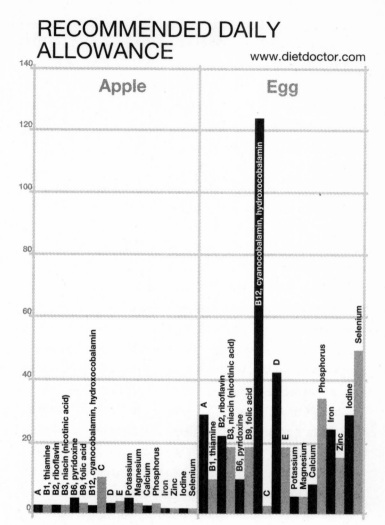

gain. Increased body weight results in decreased insulin sensitivity, which is bad.

Fruit is just about as bad as regular white sugar, which has about the same ratio of glucose and fructose. Many people insist that fruit is still good for you, because it's natural and contains a lot of other healthy nutrients. I'm saying that eating fruit is not worth it to get those "other healthy nutrients". These days, fruits contain extremely small amounts of vitamins and minerals. Compare fruit with eggs, for example; the difference is staggering. The following diagram shows a comparison of the nutritional content of 100g (3.5 oz) of apple and 100g (3.5 oz) egg.

Fruit is also said to contain dietary fibre, making it good for the digestion and intestines. We'll return to that in a moment

Starch

So, it's the glucose in our food that presents the danger. In that case, getting well would be a simple case of not touching the sugar in the sugar bowl or the fruit in the fruit bowl. As it turns out, it's more complicated than that. We still have this sinister character known as *starch*. Starch is a wolf in sheep's clothing. Or a Trojan horse, if you prefer. Starch is often thought to be a slow carb, which should somehow be better for our bodies.

So, what is this starch, really? Starch is made up of glucose molecules in rows or bunches. Increasingly often, we hear about starch as "sugar chains", which is a very good name as it perfectly describes exactly what starch is. The word "starch" sounds pretty okay, leading us to think about stiff shirt collars – not sky-high blood sugar levels.

Starch is present in grain foods such as bread, pizza and

pasta. Rice and potatoes also contain starch. So what's so tricky about starch? For one, starch doesn't taste sweet! Imagine a wheat cracker. It's not at all sweet, it tastes more like sawdust. So we easily imagine that it's good for you. But this is definitely not the case. Before you've even swallowed it, the starch starts to get chopped up into sugar molecules, which you can taste if you keep chewing for a while. When the sugar chains continue into the body, glucose molecules are freed from one another and, before you know it, blood sugar levels are up and away. Quite disappointing after you've eaten something that isn't sweet at all.

Fibre

I've already made some casual references to fibre. Dietary fibre is part of the carbohydrate family, but it's a type of carbohydrate that the body can't metabolise in the usual way. Only the intestinal bacteria can digest fiber. When bacteria digest fibre, gases form in the gut. One common result from eating fibre is bloating and flatulence – it just makes you fart. Anyone who begins to follow THE SCANDINAVIAN DIET model recommended in this book will notice soon enough that the flatulence disappears. The fibre found in grain is the most irritating to the body. Soluble fibre (such as fruit fibre) is less irritating to the stomach and intestines.

People who often get indigestion generally benefit enormously by phasing fibre out of their diet.

How much sugar does the body need?

You'll probably be told that sugar is essential for brain function. Some parts of the brain need glucose, this is true. So what happens if one does not eat sugar or starch? As far as the brain is concerned, not much at all. The brain will go about its business and use sugar where and when it needs it. The body is actually designed to synthesise glucose using fat or protein.

If someone is starving, the body will even break down muscle to make glucose. Fat is easier to carry around, so the body tries to save it as long as possible. THE SCANDINAVIAN DIET does not "starve" one, but the diet does not include much sugar or starch. People on THE SCANDINAVIAN DIET eat protein, which is used to make sugar. Muscles are actually not harmed. Fatty acids are the fuel for the synthesis.

This means that if you don't eat sugar and starch, your blood sugar will not surge out of control. At the same time, fat is burned to make the modest amounts of sugar that you actually need. By-products from this process are called ketones, and ketones can actually be used as fuel in those parts of the brain that don't require glucose, and by muscles – including the heart. It has been said that the heart and brain function 25% better running on ketones.

Is this not brilliant? THE SCANDINAVIAN DIET helps keep blood sugar at a lower level while simultaneously burning off body fat and helping the heart and brain work better!

One might ask if a sugar and starch-free diet could cause blood sugar levels to sink too low? Low blood sugar is not good, either. Of course, our bodies are designed to deal with this situation. When blood sugar goes down past a certain level, the pancreas secretes an enzyme called glucagon. Glucagon's job is to signal the liver to start synthesising sugar – so-called gluconeogenesis. For a type 2 diabetic, this means that the body is adjusting blood sugar levels to a comfortable level on its own. This is by far much kinder to the body, as opposed to constantly being at war with itself (which is what happens when you eat sugar and starch, elevating blood sugar, and then combating that with insulin, which promotes fat storage). High blood sugar and high insulin cause injury to the body due to inflammation. Eating according to THE SCANDINAVIAN DIET model will prevent this war. The body will be at peace.

Charlotte Erlanson-Albertsson sheds light on several interesting facts about carbohydrates in her book *Appetite regulation in health and disease*. For example, our fat reserves can last for two months, while carbohydrate stores only last 24 hours. This may mean that humans are basically designed to use fat as an energy source.

Adding sugar to fat reduces the satiated feeling compared to fat alone. Imagine eating a large oatmeal cookie that contains plenty of both sugar and fat, and compare it to eating the same number of calories of butter.

It's easy to trick that feeling of being full. Even after a three-course meal, you still have room for a sweet dessert. It goes down almost of its own accord. You would certainly have a harder time managing a slice of ham – even though the sweet dessert and a slice of ham contain the same number of calories.

How did we treat diabetes before?

If we open the Nordic Family Almanac from 1917 and look up "Diabetes", we see that the disease is "the inability of the organism to completely or partially digest the carbohydrates consumed in foodstuff or synthesised during metabolism". We were absolutely on the right track here. No explanation is needed regarding the ingested carbohydrates, but for carbohydrates synthesised by metabolic enzymes, we refer to glucose produced after ingesting more protein than needed.

Diabetes was classified as either "severe" or "mild". The severe sort is what we today know as type 1 diabetes, whereas the mild variant is type 2 diabetes. The mild form was described as "a slight reduction of carbohydrates in the diet causes the disappearance of sugar from the urine". Regarding the severe variant, the contemporary wisdom was that "only after complete elimination of carbohydrates from the diet, or first after concurrent reduction of protein as well."

This is exactly what THE SCANDINAVIAN DIET is all about. Reduce the carbohydrates, replace them with non-blood sugar-elevating fat and be careful not to eat too much protein.

I can tell you a story about a woman who had type 2 diabetes. This happened quite a while ago, when diabetics had to pay for their own insulin. They could, however, get a prescription for alcohol at half the price. This particular woman did not want to waste money on insulin, so she made sure to get most of her daily energy intake in the form of fat. The man who told me this story added that he thought it was nauseating to watch her slicing pork rind. In any case, that's how she managed to avoid the need for insulin. Alcohol lowers the blood sugar levels by reducing the liver's ability to produce and secrete sugar when needed. This home remedy wasn't completely wrong, judging by her lifespan. I can't remember exactly when she was born, but it should have been around the time of the American Civil War. In any case, she died in the 1960s at the age of 102. Replacing carbohydrates with fat, which does not elevate blood sugar, can in other words save a diabetic from a premature death.

I happened to come across a book from 1926, entitled: "On the treatment of diabetes (also with insulin)" by professor Karl Petrén. The author presented the conclusion that diabetes was a metabolic disturbance, characterised by the inability of the body to utilise sugar at a normal rate. Karl Petrén's words regarding the treatment of diabetes: *only in this way can it be successfully treated, and that is by the choice of a proper diet, that is by adhering to certain limitations regarding the diet. In this way, improvement can be achieved. By improvement I mean that the relevant symptoms of the disease disappear."* These are strong words, indeed. Further down, Petrén states that *"improvements can, however, also be then observed in that the weakness of the pancreas, that is, reduction of its internal secretion to the blood (production of insulin), is partially reversed."* This would indicate that diabetes can actually be reversed. This is in stark contrast to what is stated in contemporary books, which imply that a diabetic must follow the so-called "natural course" of events and succumb to a disease that continually and increasingly destroys their health. In the past, they left the door open for improvement.

This sounds exciting, so we continue: *"Seemingly, any of these types of improvement can only be achieved by subjecting oneself to certain restrictions in the diet, and the outlook for persistent improvement can only be achieved by a single means, mainly that the diabetes sufferer shall forever continue to subject himself to such restrictions regarding the diet, as in the given case are necessary. It is thusly not a simple cure, but a question of changing lifestyle."* In those days, diet was the keystone of diabetes treatment. Petrén also contemplated the question of daily calorie intake: *"If the required quantity of foodstuff is consumed, the person in question will be of stable body weight. If a larger quantity is consumed, one will under certain circumstances increase the body weight, which, however, is by no means certain; it is well-known that certain persons, who are persistently lean, may profess to a ravenous appetite. If, on the contrary, less than the required amount of foodstuff is consumed, the inevitable result is a decrease in weight."* This is an interesting paragraph. Petrén concludes that it is not at all certain that eating a lot will result in weight gain.

Advantage: metabolism?

This leads us to a complicated issue, namely: does THE SCANDINAVIAN DIET provide some sort of metabolic advantage compared to the official dietary advice? Let's take that bull by the horns.

There are several examples of people who eat extremely little, but still do not lose weight. Or, perhaps they have not lost as much weight as they should considering the caloric deficit they live with. A well-known case that provides a good example involves inhabitants of the Warsaw ghetto during WWII, who lived on a diet of only about 1700 kcal per day. Theoretically, this would result in a weight loss of about 175 kg during the two years they were trapped. Instead, their weight loss was about 15 kg. This reveals a clear error in our calorie counter. They should have burned a lot more calories. They lost about 20g per day, which translates to about 900 kcal per day instead of the normal 2500.

The calorie counter assumes that we know how much energy the body requires. That's where things become difficult.

An automobile engine being fed various amounts of fuel runs at various speeds. A lot of fuel causes the engine to run fast, whereas choking the fuel supply slows it down. The human body works the same way. It can turn off nonessential functions when the energy supply is reduced. Let's perform a thought experiment: If the body constantly requires the same amount of energy, wouldn't cutting down the energy supply

result in a rapid demise? Actually, the human body can partially shut down the immune system when energy is in short
supply.

So, how can a person on THE SCANDINAVIAN DIET
suddenly begin to lose weight, despite consuming more
energy than before? I believe that this works in the following
way: eating "more", for starters, does not necessarily mean that
you're actually eating more. Instead, if you eat enough to make
you feel full, you might perceive this to mean that you have
eaten more. In reality, you might be ingesting less energy than
before, despite not feeling any hunger pangs.

But this can't explain everything. Some studies have shown
that people who eat a larger proportion of fat lose more weight
than those consuming the same number of calories in the
form of carbohydrates. One can only speculate about what
happens in these cases, but one might propose that a generous
fat intake helps the body function as it should. For example,
there are many cases where involuntarily childless women
suddenly become pregnant after switching to THE SCANDI-
NAVIAN DIET. The energy can be put to other, good uses
that don't show up on the bathroom scales. It's hard to imagine
that the immune system's workings can be measured on a
bathroom scale, but this process also requires energy, which
means a person ingesting more calories – but in the form of
fat – can still reduce the percentage of fat in their body. They
become slimmer and also don't catch colds as often.

It is actually quite difficult to calculate how many calories
are burned. It's a lot harder than counting the calories one
eats. The only way to discover how many calories are burned

is to compare the calorie intake, then determine the change in body fat, and then recalculate this to calories. The conventional calorie counters aren't really capable of this.

Another relevant aspect is that it is easier to overeat if one eats a lot of carbohydrates. Carbohydrates act to stimulate hunger, in contrast to fat. Nor does fat elevate blood sugar, making it an excellent food for a diabetic. We have known this for quite a while, and this knowledge has been used to treat diabetics by helping them achieve a healthier blood sugar level.

Bread

Returning to Karl Petrén and his book, Petrén states that as soon as a diabetic has been diagnosed, the patient must recognise that he or she should avoid sugar for the rest of his or her life. Petrén also claimed that the diabetic should avoid any food containing flour. Except bread. Petrén explains this peculiar exception by asserting that virtually no one can come to terms with never again being able to eat bread. He does, however, suggest eliminating bread for a limited time. The author believes that, despite the fact that bread contains the most carbohydrates, humans are basically addicted to bread and can therefore not live without it.

We should nevertheless remember that we can actually live without bread. But I still remember how strange it was to not have any. We are brought up with the idea that bread is a very primal food, and that bread is good for you. And you can't deny that it is tasty. But you can quit. Once you stop eating carbohydrates, your sweet tooth also disappears after a while. The sweet tooth is actually also craving starch, not just sweets. The body knows that starch is quickly transformed into sugar, which explains our craving for bread and pasta, foods that do not taste particularly sweet. Petrén says that in order to be able to eat bread, it is extremely important to completely eliminate potatoes. He claims that potatoes are easier to avoid than bread.

Milk is also something the author urges diabetics to avoid. Cream, however, is quite okay. The higher the fat content, the better.

Petrén claims that, for psychological reasons, it's better to quit eating carbohydrates "cold turkey". Otherwise, the patient would constantly be aware of limitations in the diet. According to the doctor, after a complete and total elimination of carbohydrates, the patient can be comforted by an occasional piece of bread. I agree with him. It's difficult for a drug addict to gradually cut down to a sensible dose. It's certainly easier to quit completely and, hopefully, learn to avoid temptation.

Relief

According to Petrén's experience, success is best achieved when the diseased organ is no longer subjected to stress. A broken bone is put in a cast so that it doesn't have to bear a load. For the diabetic, reducing the carbohydrate intake reduces the load on the pancreas. In this way, the pancreas can regain its ability to produce insulin. He wrote: "*Thusly, a true recuperation from the disease is achieved.*" Consider the enormous gap between this statement and modern thinking, which states that a diabetic's health will constantly deteriorate. Today's diabetic is advised to get most of his or her energy from the carbohydrates that are making them ill.

Petrén's type 1-diabetics

In the early 20th century, type 1 diabetes was known as "the severe sugar disease". Petrén wrote that this category of illness required even greater attention to a good diet. Not only should carbohydrate intake be limited, but protein intake should also be watched carefully. Petrén had come to the conclusion that by reducing the amount of protein in the diet, the beneficial effects could be significantly greater. This is in agreement with what we know today. Excess protein is transformed into glucose, elevating the blood sugar and thereby also stimulating secretion of insulin and promoting fat storage. In order to reduce protein intake, type 1 diabetics should: *"absolutely avoid such high protein foodstuffs such as meat, fish, eggs and cheese."* Even milk was to be completely eliminated. The minimal amount of protein one might allow oneself should come from cream. One could also eat cabbage, which contains barely 2% protein. Type 1 diabetics should also consume lard, which does not elevate blood sugar. According to Petrén, this diet would only be helpful if sufficient amounts of fat were consumed. Fat should be eaten in the form of cream, lard and butter. It can also be added to coffee or tea.

Looking at the bottom line, calorie composition on this diet would be about 250 g (2200 kcal) fat, and carbohydrates and protein would be limited to 100 g (400 kcal). This means that 85% of the body's energy would come from fat. With the help of this diet, the type 1 diabetic could – for a while at least – survive without insulin.

Petrén suggests that there is no reason not to continue this dietary regimen. The only problem is that patients grow tired of it. That's why some carbohydrates and protein can be reintroduced after a while. Atkins also made use of this model. Eventually one could start to eat the food that once made one sick and obese. This way of thinking is often expressed by proponents of the GI-method.

About modern dietary advice

When the Romans sacked Carthage, the city was burned, the population was sold into slavery; the earth was ploughed and, finally, covered with salt. I think that we should do likewise with today's dietary advice to diabetics. Rather, diabetics should eat natural food that they tolerate with a minimal rise in blood sugar. This way, the diabetic need not suffer from tragic deferred complications.

Every diabetic known to me who has switched over from what the diabetes brochures call "health" food to THE SCAN-DINAVIAN DIET has experienced improved health and a reduced or eliminated need for medication and insulin. Why not give it a try? If you've read this far, you already know about the problems caused by poor blood sugar level control. This should be an incentive for change.

Did you know that there is an expression – *"adjust your diabetes"*? This involves medication and/or injecting insulin to keep blood sugar on an even keel. I really don't like that expression. It sounds like diabetes is something that you'll always have and that it should be treated with insulin. It's like you shouldn't even *try* to manage the diabetes by eating food that doesn't make it worse.

Diabetes should be treated primarily by adjusting your diet. When this approach doesn't work, medication and insulin may be used. Unfortunately it doesn't work that way these days, when newly diagnosed diabetics start to inject insulin immediately.

My first book, "Fear of Fat", was published in Swedish also as an audio book. It was very rewarding to receive feedback from people who happened to listen to the book, began to put my ideas into practice, and then either reduced or completely eliminated their medication. One of them ended up in a hospital emergency room due to his diabetes, and bought a magazine from the gift shop that contained a CD with my book. He was bored, began to listen to my audiobook and was soon afterward free from his medicine.

Of course, there are no guarantees that troublesome deferred complications won't happen, but staying on a diet that does not promote the disease is the least you can do to help avoid these problems.

What is
THE SCANDINAVIAN DIET
and how does it work?

It's time to start talking about what to do to minimise the problems of diabetes. As far as watching what you eat, it's not that difficult. Just try to eliminate carbohydrates from your diet as much as possible. Basically, carbohydrates are absent in animal- based foodstuffs. Do not eat potatoes or rice. Avoid flour like the plague. Don't even eat whole grain bread. If someone tries to tempt you with a slice, just say that you are cereal-intolerant (because you are).

To gain more insight into which foods are good for you, try to imagine what people ate before they learned how to grow grain. If we eat these original natural foods, chances are that we will be consuming things that our bodies have become used to through evolution. What would a Stone Age human choose from a supermarket?

He probably ate meat, fish, birds and eggs. We also most certainly ate nuts when we could find them, and berries when they were in season. Most modern dieticians say that we can basically eat as much fruit and vegetables as we want. They're considered to be chock-full of goodness and contain very little fat, so just go for it. The problem is that, because they contain so little fat, it's easy to eat too much and thus consume too much fructose, which promotes fat synthesis. Fruit also elevates the blood sugar level. Some people say that a diabetic should eat 15 pieces of fruit per day, but this is absolutely wrong. That's when you will need medication to keep your blood sugar down.

Getting started with THE SCANDINAVIAN DIET is a matter of eating like mankind originally ate. In the morning, eggs are an appropriate choice. A good way to limit the amount of protein is to throw some of the egg whites away. Cut the bacon into small pieces and fry it in butter; when it's done, pour the eggs over it with a little cream. Scrambled eggs will soak up the fat from the frying pan. Serve with a pat of butter, the crowning touch on an omelette from heaven …

A breakfast like this will probably get you through the

Increase in blood sugar levels (mmol/l)

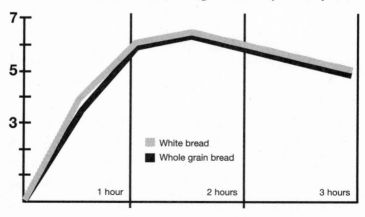

morning without needing a snack. Don't serve any whole-grain bread.

The diagram shows the blood sugar level after ingesting 50 g of carbohydrates from whole-grain and white bread, respectively. As you can see, the difference is not very great. Nevertheless, eating whole-grain bread is still widely encouraged, and many people think that whole-grain bread is a healthy choice. Diabetics should of course not eat any bread at all. There is no simpler rule of thumb, and the bread issue doesn't get any more complicated than that. Bread is starch and starch is glucose, the kind of sugar that elevates your blood sugar level.

If you can, you should pack a lunch for work because THE SCANDINAVIAN DIET-food is generally not available at cafeterias. It will take a while for THE SCANDINAVIAN DIET to gain enough popularity to make low-carb meals common on restaurant menus, but if everyone who prefers THE SCANDINAVIAN DIET makes a point of requesting low-carb dishes at cafeterias and restaurants, the owners will begin to take notice. They do want to keep their customers, and get new ones.

After a while, you might even be able to learn to skip lunch. Otherwise, a slice of cheese or some other small snack can tide you over. The craving for sweets disappears after a while, and instead of feeling full, you'll simply not be hungry. It's a strange feeling to get up from the table when you'd still like to eat some more. After a few minutes, however, you become indifferent to food and stay that way for quite a while. People in the far north of Sweden have an amusing expression, "*dumpling coma*", which most of us will recognise after having eaten way too much pizza. You won't need to feel that way ever again.

If you occasionally indulge in spirits, you'll notice that you'll need fewer drinks to get to the same relaxed state. I'm not sure exactly how that works; perhaps your body becomes rejuvenated and more sensitive to alcohol.

Lunch and dinner consist of meat, fish or poultry. If you choose a lean cut of meat, make sure to include a side of something fatty. Otherwise you'll become hungry again quite soon. There are hundreds of low-carb recipes available on the Internet, and increasingly more low-carb cookbooks are being published (just make sure they include enough fat).

To eat or not to eat

Here are a few quick reference guides to help you decide what to indulge in and what to avoid. Different people can eat different amounts of carbohydrates, but for diabetics it's extra important to cut down on them. Cream can be tricky, for example. Some people have no problem with cream, whereas others seem to be unable to lose weight. A little bit of trial and error is necessary to see what is best for you. Diabetics should try to eat no more than 20 g of carbohydrates per day, and absolutely no more than 60 g. In the beginning, keeping track of everything can be difficult, so here are some tips:

OK

Milk products

Use full-fat cream. Feta cheese is good. Butter is excellent for cooking. Blend it with seasonings as a condiment and use it for frying.

Eggs

Eggs are probably the perfect food. If you really like eggs, you might want to be careful with the egg whites, otherwise you might get too much protein.

Coconut oil

Coconut oil is perfectly good for your body. Use a little in your coffee or tea. If you're feeling a little peckish, it's often enough to have a little coconut oil to get rid of the cravings. "Veteran low-carbers" carry a small jar of coconut oil around wherever they go. In a pinch, a tablespoon can be a great substitute for lunch.

Fish

Fish is an excellent food. Herring, mackerel and salmon are fatty fish that contain lots of essential omega-3 fats. If you're having a leaner fish, smother it in a rich sauce. It's quite simple; mix some mayonnaise with full-fat sour cream and season to taste. Add as much as you feel like, you're the boss now!

Vegetables

Eat your vegetables, but don't overdo it. They aren't that nourishing, they can be expensive and some vegetables can be tricky regarding carbohydrates. Stick with those that grow above ground. This is a simple rule of thumb that works quite well. Instead of mashed potatoes, try some mashed cauliflower with a generous pat of butter. Mix in some grated Parmesan cheese and voilá! Season to taste.

Meat

Meat is an original food for the human race, which tells us that it is good. Unfortunately, animals used in modern meat production are often fed various types of feed that result in meat containing high levels of omega-6 fatty acids, which promote inflammation. Meat from organically raised animals is the best. South American beef cattle are generally grass fed, which is good.

Pork

Pork is an excellent meat. I love bacon in the morning. Unfortunately, cured bacon almost always contains glucose. Salted or pickled pork is generally a better choice for breakfast.

Poultry

Chicken is the most common poultry, and it's just fine if you liven it up with rich side dishes and sauces.

Coffee and tea

Coffee tends to raise insulin levels somewhat, so very discriminating folks will choose caffeine-free coffee. Otherwise, tea is a good alternative. Water is best with meals. Keep a jug in the refrigerator; it's tastier than water straight from the tap.

Nuts

Small amounts of nuts are OK, but that's it. 100 g of nuts contains about 10 g of carbohydrates, so if you want to have less than 20 g of carbohydrates per day, don't overdo the nuts.

Rich sauces

Absolutely! Be careful, though, to avoid those artificial powder mixes from the supermarket. Make homemade Béarnaise sauce instead.

Do not eat

Dairy products

The dairy product to avoid is milk. Moderate amounts are not that bad, but milk is often drunk by the glass, which causes a blood sugar peak. A glass of milk can elevate blood sugar just as much as several glucose tablets.

Watch out for rich yoghurts. Check the label for carbohydrate content, and see what you have room for in your "carb budget".

Fruit

Don't!

Grain products

Grain products can consist of various forms of bread, pasta, porridge, gruel, breakfast flakes and muesli. These products contain starch, which significantly elevates blood sugar.

Potatoes

Potatoes grow underground, and are therefore among the plants you should not eat. Nor should you eat carrots or anything else growing underground.

Rice

Rice contains a lot of starch, which makes it a no-no. Rice cakes are also rice, and contain about 80% carbohydrates.

Sweet beverages

It goes without saying that sweetened beverages are no longer on the menu. Not even artificially sweetened ones. They can still stimulate insulin secretion because the body is fooled into thinking that it's "sugar time". The sugar fails to show up, and blood sugar levels decrease due to the released insulin. Fat reserves are locked down and the body prepares to store even more fat, which is convenient as you will soon be hungry due to the decreased blood sugar level. You will eat and grow fat. Try to wean yourself from your sweet tooth. This is a significant victory.

If you are on medication that lowers blood sugar (Glucophage/Metformin do *not* belong to this category) or if you take insulin, it's extremely important to monitor your blood sugar levels when switching over to THE SCANDINAVIAN DIET. Your blood sugar levels will tend to return to normal on THE SCANDINAVIAN DIET, and insulin or medication that lowers blood sugar levels may cause them to dip dangerously low.

Check your blood sugar carefully when switching over to THE SCANDINAVIAN DIET!

You can find additional resources on the Internet about the carbohydrate content of various foods.

Can my symptoms disappear?

Type 1

I met a man who had suffered from type 1 diabetes for about 15 years. He had experimented with a low-carb diet, and in that way managed to avoid insulin injections on some days. He belonged to the group that still had some insulin production, and that's why, by controlling his intake of carbohydrates and protein, he could maintain his blood sugar level at a normal level without insulin injections.

In other words, patients who still produce some insulin can in some cases manage their diabetes without additional insulin, as incredible as it may seem.

Research is under way on vaccines that can slow down the destruction of beta cells (which synthesise insulin), providing hope for newly diagnosed type 1 diabetics. Such a vaccine may even help people with a weak but still active insulin production, even if they've had diabetes for a long time. We can only hope that this research will continue, and that the companies conducting this research aren't bought up and shut down. Unfortunately, diabetics are a cash cow for Big Pharma (the pharmaceutical industry). It would be a huge disaster for them if the steady stream of new type 1 diabetics dried up. Patients spend their entire lives buying insulin, glucose measurement equipment, testing strips and other accessories.

Type 2

Today many people suffering from diabetes have success-fully eliminated insulin injections. Many more have been able to reduce their medication, and quite a few can manage their disease simply by switching to a diet that only minimally elevates blood sugar. It's easy to choose food that doesn't elevate blood sugar that much. Still, many people have trouble giving up their favourites like bread and potatoes. I know that many people perceive bread as one of life's necessities, and this is understandable. It tastes good, and you can put lots of good things on it. It also provides quick energy by elevating the blood sugar level. But bread is not at all good for people with metabolic disturbances. Saying no to bread is a signifi-cant victory. Phasing out potatoes, pasta and rice is an addi-tional huge step to improved health. Succeeding with this means that one has slowed down the progression of diabetes as much as possible, and one can often get by with no medical treatment and a healthy blood sugar level. It's both simple and elegant.

Can diabetes be cured?

Type 1

The problem with type 1 diabetes is that the pancreas has stopped producing enough insulin. Today, whole-pancreas transplants are possible, but it's still both unusual and risky. One alternative to whole-pancreas transplants is to transplant only the insulin-producing cells, which is done by injecting them into the liver. This is a relatively safe method, but after five years, about 90% of these patients must resume insulin injections. Injected cell islands successively die off, and it is believed that this is due to poor oxygenation, as the newly generated blood vessels adjacent to them cannot transport enough oxygen.

A substance known as amyloid also appears to prevent transplanted cells from functioning properly. Amyloid is generated as a result of stress, and one way to increase cell survival and function is to reduce the stress they are subjected to during transplantation.

The availability of functioning cell islands from humans is insufficient to treat every type 1 diabetic. To solve this problem, experiments are being performed with porcine (pig) cells.

As far as I know, these cells have only been transplanted to apes thus far, but pig insulin works perfectly in lowering blood sugar levels in humans. So it is possible that cell islands from pigs could also be transplanted.

Type 2

There is, in fact, an operation that can cure type 2 diabetics or in any case, normalise blood sugar levels without medication or insulin. Strangely enough, no one really knows how it works. It was discovered during gastric surgery. Doctors noticed that surgery relieved diabetes symptoms. What happens is that the duodenum is no longer connected to the stomach in the usual way.

One theory proposes that the disconnection of the duodenum from the stomach causes abnormal signalling from the duodenum, the factor which might cause diabetes. This explanation is called the *anti-incretin theory*. It's based on the idea that incretin – a hormone secreted in the intestine – stimulates insulin secretion. Too much insulin lowers the blood sugar level too much. Excessively low blood sugar levels are dangerous, so the body has protective mechanisms. This particular protective mechanism could be a type of anti-incretin mechanism. Healthy humans have a stable balance between incretin and anti-incretin systems, leading to a proper and stable blood sugar level.

It's possible that, in some people, the duodenum produces too much anti-incretin. As a result, insulin secretion is reduced and the body finally succumbs to diabetes.

Cells in diabetics are less sensitive to insulin than in others, but according to this theory, disconnection of the duodenum would prevent its reduction of insulin secretion, thus curing the diabetes.

This may sound attractive, but the downside is that surgery is always risky. Unnecessary surgery should always be avoided. In addition, not enough is known about the long-term health effects of manipulating the duodenum. There may be other effects, perhaps even worse than diabetes.

Hopefully, research on the function of the duodenum will continue, and more specific knowledge about the effects of disconnecting it from the stomach will be obtained. This could lead to the development of a less invasive procedure, or perhaps to the discovery of drugs that would have the same effect as a disconnected duodenum. We'll see what happens. In any case, this is exciting and we hope that a real diabetes cure is not too far down the road.

Increasing the effect

There are methods other than adjusting the diet which can reduce symptoms, especially for type 2 diabetics. Physical exertion reduces the need for insulin in order for sugar to enter muscle cells. Because hard-working cells need more sugar, their insulin resistance is lowered. As a result, blood sugar levels tend towards normal values.

Increase insulin sensitivity by exercising

Today's diabetes patients are generally encouraged to consume most of their energy in the form of carbohydrates. With this diet, insulin injections are necessary to keep blood sugar levels under control. Injecting insulin is not particularly accurate, especially compared to the body's own dose adjustment mechanisms. As a rule, too much insulin is administered, resulting in storage instead of burning of fat.

As the patient becomes increasingly obese, higher doses of insulin are required, with increased body weight as a result. Greater body weight leads to poorer insulin sensitivity, which is in turn treated by increased doses of insulin. This natural course of events is considered to be inevitable and normal. I've even heard it referred to as "the insulin course of events", which is much more accurate, because it's especially linked to increased insulin dosage.

Proponents of the "natural course of events" model say that a diabetic's condition *MUST* worsen and require increased doses of medication. Unfortunately, patients who try to reverse this downward spiral and reduce their need for insulin are often met with suspicion by diabetes treatment professionals. By meekly following directions and proceeding along the negative spiral, long-term negative effects will inevitably appear. Problems with the eyes, feet, kidneys and cardio-vascular system will arise.

Let's look at what happens in a typical diabetes treatment centre today:

1. You're encouraged to eat lots of carbohydrates.
2. The more carbohydrates you eat, the higher your blood sugar will become.
3. The higher your blood sugar becomes, the more insulin is required.
4. The more insulin you have in your body, the fatter you will become.
5. The fatter you become, the more insulin is required, and the last resort is injecting insulin with a needle. Go back to step 4.

And so on and so on, and the only ones who benefit from this are the people who produce and sell insulin. Diabetics are a wonderful cash cow for Big Pharma. We estimate that there are 300 million diabetics worldwide, and this is a group that drug manufacturers are extremely reluctant to lose. It's been said that more people make a living from diabetes than die from it. In his book "Side Effects: Death. Confessions of a Pharma-Insider", German author John Virapen writes:

> *"Once again we're discussing a drug not only known for its questionable efficacy, but also for its side effects. There are primarily two major side effects: weight gain and increased risk of developing diabetes. Patients who experience these side effects require additional medication – such as insulin."*

If you don't want to spend unnecessary sums of your own as well as taxpayers' money on diabetes medication, you should try to find that positive spiral that will help you escape the grip of the sugar disease.

Richard K. Bernstein's training

Physician Richard K. Bernstein describes a diabetic's optimal exercise regimen in his book "Dr. Bernsteis's Diabetes Solution". According to Bernstein, insulin sensitivity is dependent on the ratio between visceral fat (fat in and around the gut region) and muscle mass. In other words, a trim waist and well-developed muscles indicate a higher insulin sensitivity. Good sensitivity to insulin means that less insulin is needed. Less insulin coursing through the body means lowered fat storage. The less fat that is stored in the body, the higher the insulin sensitivity, and once again, less insulin is required. One simply gets better. For once, we have a positive spiral. Compare this spiral to what happens in our standard model for diabetes treatment (see above, 1-5).

Bernstein describes various types of muscle fibres. Some muscle fibres are used during light exertion over a prolonged time, such as when we walk or ride a bicycle. The workload is not especially great when these fibres are active. These fibres use something called *aerobic* metabolism, where less glucose but much oxygen is utilised.

There is yet another type of muscle fibre that is used during strenuous exertion. These are known as *anaerobic* fibres. They can support a much greater load, but don't have the same stamina. This work uses a lot of glucose and hardly any oxygen.

Now hold on ... lots of glucose is needed to perform strenuous tasks ... A diabetic's problem is an overly high blood sugar level. So this would mean that if we work the muscles that use anaerobic metabolism, we could transfer sugar from the blood, where it causes problems, to muscle cells that help us do the heavy lifting. How ingenious! The harmful blood sugar disappears during harmless exertion such as lifting a barbell or some other heavy object.

And on top of that, the body knows that lots of sugar is used during strenuous exertion, so it will create more glucose transporters from blood to muscle cells, because it's important that the cells can quickly receive enough sugar. This means that strenuous physical exertion improves transport of sugar from the blood into the muscles not only during exertion, but afterwards as well.

Bernstein's experience is that it takes about 14 days of intensive training to significantly improve insulin sensitivity. If that seems daunting, we can comfort ourselves knowing that the effect lasts for 14 days after training stops. In other words, taking a break for a week isn't that tragic. A type 2 diabetic who takes insulin must therefore increase insulin dosage 14 days after stopping training.

A few months are usually required, however, before the gradual improvement of insulin sensitivity from the improved muscle mass- to visceral fat ratio is noticeable. However, the daily training needed to develop these muscles affects insulin sensitivity much sooner.

Anaerobic muscle fibres produce lactic acid when exercised. We notice this as pain or cramps in that muscle, and it soon loses all its strength. When the strain stops, the lactic acid dissipates within a few seconds. In order for this glucose-craving muscle fibre to crave even more glucose and be less sensitive to lactic acid-induced pain, it needs to be developed. It develops by becoming larger and synthesising more glucose transporters on the cell surface.

To stimulate development of the muscle fibre, you must exercise it strenuously and intensively. Then you experience lactic acid pain. Lactic acid can be compared to a receipt, proving that you have worked the muscle properly. Unfortunately, lactic acid doesn't persist very long. The pain and your instincts both tell you to quickly let go of the barbell and regain use of your arm. There are ways, however, to prolong the elevated lactic acid level and keep the muscle working longer. Normally, a bodybuilder will start with lighter weights and then successively increase the load until the maximum is reached. This is not really the best way. Because lactic acid is involved in muscle fibre development, it's most effective to work with the maximum load immediately.

The method

After warming up, begin with a weight that you can only lift/pull 3 to 4 times. The trick here is to go through the motions slowly. Lifting should take about 7 seconds, whereas returning to resting position should take about 5 seconds. After 3-4 lifts or pulls, you should reduce the weight so that you can do 3-4 lifts/pulls again as soon as possible, before the muscle has had time to rest up. Keep going until you've done a total of 20 reps. Now you're finished with that muscle group for the day. Or, more correctly, for at least 48 hours. What actually happens is that the muscle cell is depleted for the next 24 hours, after which it grows/develops during the 24 hours following that. That's why it's not very sensible to work out the same muscle group every day, because you end up in a mix of depletion/growth of the muscle.

Don't make the exercises too easy. You won't need very heavy weights, because the motion should be performed slowly. When you feel the lactic acid, you'll know that you've got it right.

Set up your training schedule to exercise different muscle

groups during each session. For example, train the legs and abdomen on day one, back muscles on day two and shoulders, chest and arms on day three. That way, your muscles will have time to develop between sessions.

After your first session, you'll most certainly become acquainted with fibrils. Fibrils, part of the muscle cells, need to recuperate and become stronger after exertion. This is almost always accompanied by muscle ache, which is usually at its worst 48 hours after exercise. You are experiencing delayed onset muscle soreness. It's not harmful to continue your training while the muscles are sore. But it's no fun, either.

Training in this way is very effective. You can limit your sessions in the gym to 15 to 20 minutes. While you're there, you'll probably see people casually lifting weights that don't seem to require much effort. One might wonder what the benefit is, aside from socialising. As far as I'm concerned, hard and intensive training is the right way. A short time with the maximum load gives results. While exercising, your muscles will hurt and that's how you'll know you're working hard enough. "No pain – no gain" is true enough. You'll be panting like a dog when you hit the showers, especially after a leg workout. And you weren't even in the gym very long!

If you haven't been doing strenuous workouts for a while, you should get a medical exam before you begin. A diabetic with weak retinal blood vessels can sustain eye injury after sudden exertion.

Type 2 diabetics have the most to gain from muscle development training, as they have decreased insulin sensitivity. Type 1 diabetics generally do not, but who would mind feeling a bit more "ripped"? And what diabetic would shun the opportunity to get rid of some sugar from the bloodstream into the muscles?

So, what about the typically recommended types of exercise? Walking, bicycling, swimming and so on? This kind of exercise is certainly not harmful, but it's not really useful for weight loss or controlling blood sugar. The reason is that during so-called aerobic training, muscles use lots of oxygen but not that much sugar. Nor does it build up muscle mass, either. Aerobic training doesn't help with insulin sensitivity in type 2 diabetics very much. The saying goes that food puts on the pounds and exercise takes off the ounces. So if you're looking to lose weight, low intensity training is not very effective. You'll need to train for hours each day in order to see any effect.

On the contrary, transfer of sugar from the blood to the muscles is much more effective during high-intensity workouts, resulting in a decreased need for insulin (which promotes fat storage). That's how intense exercise lowers blood sugar and trims your body.

Don't eat like experts tell you to

I've been browsing through a Swedish book by Charlotte Erlanson-Albertsson, "Appetite regulation". She writes that "many small meals provide an effective way to derail the body's satiation signals". This is particularly interesting because we've been taught to eat three meals and three healthy snacks a day. Both the Swedish Diabetes Association and the Swedish Heart and Lung Association teach us this in their brochure "Good food for everyone". But according to the author of "Appetite Regulation", satiation signals are fooled, resulting in increased hunger pangs. There is even a fashionable diet called "the 3-hour diet".

Official dietary advice for diabetics and healthy people is quite peculiar. It's hard to believe that those responsible for this advice have a clue about how the body actually works. A diabetic is advised to consume about 50–60% of the daily energy intake in the form of carbohydrates. That's almost the amount of carbohydrates a sumo wrestler eats to become as massive as possible. Sumo wrestlers commonly contract diabetes after a while in the business. And that's what they're telling us to eat …

If you visit a website that is suppose to be giving good advice to diabetics, you may encounter the following:

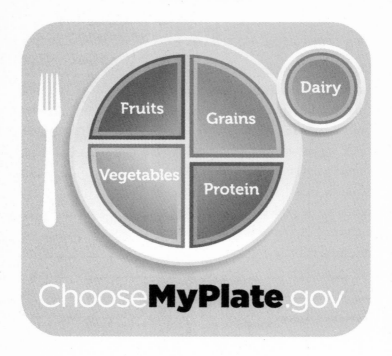

ChooseMyPlate.gov

A healthy meal for a diabetic would consist of almost half a plate of macaroni (starch that is converted to glucose), maybe a third vegetables (mostly water and starch), and about a quarter of "real" food. They also think that milk is healthy, although it contains lactose (glucose linked to galactose). They also recommend bread (starch, which is converted to glucose) and fruit (glucose linked to fructose, which is stored as fat). It's definitely not easy to keep blood sugar levels in check with this kind of advice. With friends like that, who needs enemies? Keeping your blood sugar level under control with a diet like that requires medication. We've strayed quite a way from the kind of treatment I touched upon earlier, described in the Nordic family almanac from 1917.

Losing weight obviously requires burning the calories you eat, and then some. A high carbohydrate intake builds up fat due to increased insulin levels, making it extremely difficult to lose weight. A high carbohydrate diet also makes it harder to avoid eating often and too much. The blood sugar increase is followed by a blood sugar decrease, with the resulting hunger pangs.

In other words, you have to starve yourself if you eat a low-fat diet. On a starvation diet, nonessential bodily functions are turned off, muscle mass is used for energy and the immune systems suffers. A low carbohydrate diet typically leads to a spontaneous reduction of energy intake.

Sugar addiction

Switching to a low carbohydrate diet can become quite complicated if sugar addiction is in the picture. The sugar addict isn't necessarily crazy about sugar, spooning it straight from the sugar bowl. By now you know that sugar is also present in whole wheat bread, pasta and potatoes. So a person who just loves potatoes might not understand that they're actually addicted to sugar. Completely eliminating bread, pasta and potatoes can be a daunting task.

One might rightly ask if sugar addiction actually exists. Apparently, it's a sensitive issue, and this kind of research is not permitted in Sweden. Various problems would probably surface if sugar addiction were an officially recognised condition. Doctors could prescribe disability leave, and special treatment centres would help "detox" sugar addicts. Children might be removed from households where parents are suffering from this chemical dependency.

You might think that this is a gross exaggeration, but there are cases of people shoplifting, running red lights and exhibiting other bizarre behaviour to satisfy a sugar craving.

Sweden's foremost expert on the subject is Bitten Jonsson.

She's written books and held seminars on sugar addiction, now mostly for healthcare professionals. According to Bitten Jonsson, health-care workers in the United States are far more advanced regarding recognition of sugar addiction as a disease. Sadly, research in Sweden is at a standstill. Charlotte Erlanson-Albertsson knows full well what happens if one tries to study this taboo subject in Sweden. In her book "Belöning och beroende" (Reward and dependency), she relates her experiences trying to obtain grants for research on whether sugar addiction exists or not.

In her experiments, animals given a sugar solution began to display dependency-like behaviour after three weeks. Consumption of the sugar solution increased successively. A threefold increase was observed after one week. Shivering and shaking was observed in the animals for 12 hours after being deprived of the sugar solution. They also displayed anxiety symptoms, refusing to forage or leave their enclosure.

Changes similar to those observed with high doses of alcohol or nicotine were seen in the animal's brains. The sugar solution had triggered a reward system, including compulsive behaviour and raised tolerance.

Dr. Erlanson-Albertsson wanted to investigate whether similar changes could be observed in humans. Her goal was to recruit 20 human volunteers who considered themselves to be addicted to sugar. The volunteers would need to abstain from sugar for six weeks. The fact that sugar is also present in starch is beside the point here, because the response from the authorities is the relevant issue (I'm not sure if the volunteers would be required to abstain from starch).

It doesn't matter now. The ethical review board refused to grant permission for this experiment. In other words, she was not allowed to let a few people not eat sugar for six weeks! This decision was appealed to the central research ethical committee, where most appeals are successful. In this case, however, it was still no go. The committee justified their decision with the opinion that experimental subjects would be subjected to cruel treatment if sugar was removed from their diet, and the experiment would most likely lead to feelings of guilt and self-loathing!

My take on this is that dependence is like an empty jar that needs to be filled with something. Or perhaps like an empty sack. Useless unless you fill it with something. What you actually put in it might be a bit of this or a bit of that. Dr. Erlanson-Albertsson later confirmed that women in a Swedish correctional facility were using sugar as a substitute for earlier drug use. Dependence was thus maintained, and it triggered the same reward systems that various other drugs had previously triggered. Fatty snacks did not provide the same level of comfort. Instead, fatty snacks induced nausea; the reward came only from sweets.

Not everyone can get the sugar "monkey off their back" so easily. People can be divided into two categories. In the first category, sugar is pleasant until it becomes too sweet, at which point it becomes disgusting. The second category has no limit for "too" sweet.

Having a predisposition for sweets can be hazardous to your health. In her book, Dr. Erlanson-Albertsson suggests a test to see which category one belongs to. Take two glasses and fill them with about three fluid ounces (90ml) of water. Dissolve one sugar cube in the first glass and six sugar cubes in a second glass. If both of them taste about as good, you belong to the group of people with no limits regarding sweetness. As we know, sugar is not only refined white cane sugar, but is also contained in starch. This is much trickier, because that doesn't even taste sweet on your tongue. So a craving for sugar can be satisfied with macaroni or bread, without your even knowing that it's a craving for sugar.

Children are especially vulnerable to sugar addiction. Sugar provides the functional basis for a reward system. Sugar is present in so many products today. Think about all the yoghurt pots with nutritional seals of approval, not to mention all the sweets and carbonated drinks. After this reward system is established, the next drug in line will be working with the same system for which sugar paved the way.

Bitten Jonsson has related how alcoholics can suppress their alcohol cravings for long periods if supplied with enough sugar. My own homespun theory is that this is how binge drinking works. For a while, a binge drinker can get by on sugar (starch), but eventually falls off the wagon and returns to alcohol for a while.

Addiction can have many facets, and it doesn't need to be something one consumes. Another example of behavioural dependency is religion. There are numerous examples of alcoholics who have freed themselves from alcohol dependency by being "born-again". Yet another is sex addiction. Dependencies can thus be replaced by other dependencies, but becoming completely rid of them is extremely difficult, and requires taking one day at a time and struggling through it. The core message in the 1972 Swedish comedy, "*The Man Who Quit Smoking*", is that "the sum of our vices is constant", and this seems quite plausible.

Because this book is about diabetes, we cannot exhaustively explore sugar addiction; numerous references and resources on the Internet are available to anyone wanting more information.

Children with diabetes

Diabetic children are generally of type 1, although adult onset diabetes, as type 2 is often referred to, is now being observed more often in younger individuals. Even children can manage without carbohydrates, though they're often less sensitive to their negative effects than adults. Because children are more active, the problems are not as severe. I believe that even children with diabetes should minimise their carbohydrate intake. Insulin dosage can be reduced with a low-carb diet. High blood sugar must be countered with a large insulin injection, and the more insulin that is administered, the harder it is to adjust blood sugar levels. Small elevations in blood sugar lead to small doses of insulin, thus minimising the risk of over- or under-dosing. Of course, this also applies to adults.

"Doesn't she ever cry?"

While we're on the subject, let me tell you about a 16 month old girl who was raised with THE SCANDINAVIAN DIET. The staff at the local Child Health Centre would definitely throw a fit if they knew what the child had been given to eat, so this family will remain anonymous. Here's what they told me:

Not only did the child live on THE SCANDINAVIAN DIET all her life, but her mother did likewise during the pregnancy and while breast-feeding. For breakfast, the girl generally had one or two scrambled eggs, six or seven tablespoons of cream with ham, roast beef or sausage mixed in. She washed this down with green tea with some cream. For a snack, she had rolls of ham and cheese with butter or bits of traditional Swedish sausage.

Lunch would be basically pot luck, but as a rule it consisted of beef, salmon or chicken with a rich sauce. They used to serve a little rice with it, but not anymore. She also gets some vegetables such as cauliflower, carrots etc.

Dinner was whatever the adults were having, also according to THE SCANDINAVIAN DIET of course, and the yolks of one or two soft-boiled eggs.

Bedtime snacks were a compromise: organically produced porridge with some butter (Dad insisted on porridge). The hot liquid was cooled with an equal volume of cream. In other words, a world of fat.

Basically, the girl's staple diet consisted of organically produced eggs ever since she was weaned. She had been eating like this since she was six months old. At eleven months, she stopped suckling on her own accord.

The little girl sleeps very well at night. Usually, 12 hours. Bedtime is no problem. Bath, bed and sleep. When she wakes, she's usually happy and not in any rush to eat breakfast, because she's still nourished from the previous evening. The parents think it's great not to have to stress and make breakfast for her at five o'clock in the morning.

She's always been stable, content and calm. During her first year, the parents often heard the question: "Doesn't she ever cry?"

In all fairness, it should be noted that the girl doesn't always eat as much as I've described above.

Measuring your body

There are several methods for measuring the body to reveal conditions like obesity. The most common one is to weigh yourself. Measuring the pressure that the soles of your feet exert upon the earth's crust seems irrelevant to me. I'm not alone in my heresy, and other methods have been devised.

BMI

One that is in common use today is BMI- Body Mass Index. Calculating BMI is a bit complicated. Using metric measurements, the weight is divided by the square of the height. If our test subject is 170 cm tall and weighs 80 kg, the BMI then becomes (80 kg / (1.7 x 1.7)) = 27.7. Aside from the tedious arithmetic, it's a pretty worthless measurement, because muscle mass is penalised. Ex-governor of California Arnold Schwarzenegger had a BMI of 29.7 in his prime; in other words, seriously overweight and bordering on obese.

WHTR

A simpler model is WHTR – Waist to Height Ratio. If the waist measurement is less than half of the height in centimetres, you're not lugging around too much fat. This model doesn't penalise you for muscle mass. If the waist measurement in our example was 85 cm, that would be about 50% of the height.

Arnold could have permitted himself a measurement of 188 / 2, that is, up to 94 cm. Now his waist measured just 81 cm, which isn't bad. That was then. Today, who knows?

Waist to Height Ratio 1/2

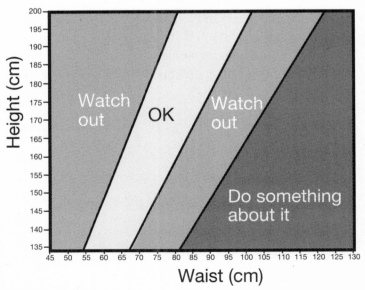

MMI, Muscular Mass Index

I raised the problematic nature of these values with my ana-lytical friend Erik Edlund, who has become very interested in diabetes and diet. He immediately began to try to devise a better method. He came up with a formula where the weight is divided by the square of the waist measurement (in metres). Our fictitious subject would thus have an index of 110, indi-cating quite a muscular figure. (80 kg/(0.85 waist x 0.85 waist). If he had had a waist measurement of 100 cm – in other words a bit of a paunch – the MMI index would be 80/1 = 80; a lower value in other words. The higher the value, the more muscular and lean the body. This method is by no means complete, but I wouldn't be surprised if something along the lines of our MMI index will soon replace BMI; nearly everyone considers the BMI a poor description of the real world.

Arnold Schwarzenegger would have had a value of 160(!), calculated as 105 kg/(0.81 x 0.81).

What are the objections?

Today's strategies for reducing diabetics' blood sugar levels focus primarily on losing weight. Decreased body weight will increase insulin sensitivity. This is all well and good, except for one problem. Because we have decided that eating fat makes you fat and carbohydrates are good for you, diabetics can only lose weight by virtually starving themselves. This method has never worked on volunteers. The paltry amount one is allowed to eat consists mostly of carbohydrates, and as we well know, carbohydrates raise the blood sugar, after which we need insulin to lower it again. Insulin can also shut down fat metabolism, and even promote fat storage. You know this by now.

You must also have realised by now that this is not a sensible way of dealing with the problem. As long as you stick to the starvation diet, you can lose weight – even if it's mainly *muscle mass* that is lost. During the process, it seems all good and well. But later, you inevitably tire of being constantly hungry and craving food, so most people resume eating again. This often entails having sandwiches and other goodies, and soon the lost weight is regained. This weight increase now consists mainly of *fat*. That's how one can deplete the body of muscle, and because a high carbohydrate diet leads to fat retention, losing weight next time is all the more difficult. Successfully losing weight time and again only to regain it soon enough is known as *yo-yo dieting*.

So what objections might one encounter as a diabetic when trying to self-medicate with natural food?

Bad for your heart

It's generally considered dangerous for diabetics to eat fat, as the risk for cardiovascular disease increases. This could be linked to the cholesterol hypothesis. Since the 1950's, we generally assumed that saturated fat increases cholesterol levels, which in turn increases the risk of heart disease. A man by the name of Ancel Keys was responsible for the studies behind this theory. This research has long been recognised as fraudulent, but the conclusions still haunt us as truths. For those who want to read more about this fantastic story, I recommend Uffe Ravnskov's book "Fett och kolesterol är hälsosamt", (Fat and cholesterol are good for you) Optimal publishers, 2008.

How well-founded are these warnings? There are, of course, no guarantees against heart attack or stroke. We also know that diabetics are already predisposed to contract these diseases compared to the average person. But what happens if a diabetic abandons mainstream thinking, cuts down on carbohydrates and eats more fat instead?

According to current wisdom, we should eat more carbohydrates and less fat. It is said that more fat increases the risk for cardiovascular disease. It's easy to forget that – aside from the fact that natural fat is good for you – the risks associated with high blood sugar caused by high carbohydrate intake far outweigh the benefits that might be associated with a low-fat diet.

The Karlshamn Study

One well-known study, the Karlshamn Study, convincingly demonstrates the benefits of a specific diet for type 2 diabetics. In this study, two groups of diabetics were given the choice between eating according to the "plate model" or cutting down on carbohydrates and increasing the amount of fat in the diet. After 44 months, results were observed that seem quite peculiar to those who believe Ancel Keys' data. A significant number of subjects abandoned the "plate model". Only one third of the original group of five people remained in this group. Of the five, four had suffered heart attacks, two of which were fatal. Expressed as a percentage, 80% of the group had experienced heart attacks, and 40% had died.

After 44 months, the "fat-eating" group consisted of 23 people. Of the 23, only two contracted cardiovascular disease, one of whom had a heart attack and one had a stroke. In addition, both subjects had lapsed in their diet and had begun to eat potatoes and bread again. They had also gained 5-6 kg per month. Both had also developed cardiovascular disease, even if both had survived it.

The results of this study lead us to the conclusion that a high-fat, low-carb diet presents a lower risk for diabetics. It even seems that cutting down on carbs and increasing fat intake is generally beneficial to anyone's health. Convincing you of this is precisely the aim of this book.

Cholesterol

I'm sure that everyone has heard that high cholesterol values are extremely dangerous. If one looks at the results of medical studies, no connection has been shown between cholesterol levels and atherosclerosis. In studies on elderly patients, the opposite has been demonstrated; high cholesterol values are associated with prolonged life. Pondering the ins and outs of "good" and "bad" cholesterol is apparently a waste of time.

There is, however, a ratio of ApoB to ApoA1, the so-called apolipoprotein quotient, which may be significant. There are tiny, dense lipoproteins that can lodge in the arterial walls, turn rancid and promote inflammation, resulting in a heart attack. It's interesting to note that this ratio improves with a reduced carbohydrate diet. Once again, cutting down on fat is the wrong way to go.

The brain

Many people think that carbohydrates are necessary for proper brain function. This is wrong. The amount of sugar that the brain requires is readily produced by the body using either the glycerol part of triglyceride molecules or protein. Amino acids and fatty acids suffice as starting material. Very clever, Mother Nature! When synthesising sugar, the body burns fat. This won't happen if insulin levels are too high, because the body uses sugar directly. Fat stores remain untouched, and they like to park themselves on your derrière.

Fat makes you fat

Chief physician Christer Enkvist coined the classical phrase: "It's just as silly to think that fat makes you fat as it is to think that greens turn you green". As you now know, fat does not increase blood sugar, and insulin levels do not surge, preventing fat stores from being burned. You won't burn fat with high insulin levels unless you're a professional athlete or in basic training with an elite military unit. The most efficient way to increase insulin levels is by eating carbohydrates. In this case, fat is not the solution.

True stories

To keep this book from becoming too rigid and dry, let me liven it up with some true stories of diabetics who have greatly improved their health. Thanks to everyone who's helped me and allowed me to relate their experiences with THE SCANDINAVIAN DIET.

Anders

Here is Anders' story:

> *Howdy!*
> *Thanks for a great book! "Fear of fat" gave me a new lease on life. I bought it in January 2006, when I had decided to try to lose weight. During the past 20 years, I've gained about 2 kg per year. I've always been convinced that my weight gain was caused by eating too much fat … arrrgh.*
>
> *Well, anyway, in January 2006 I began to read your book. I wasn't feeling well, and I was tired as hell. In February 2006, I went to my family doctor because I thought I had an infection that wouldn't go away. A few days later, a nurse called*

me, hysterically telling me that I had diabetes, because there was too much sugar in my urine sample. The value was about 11. This was a funny coincidence, because just as I was told about my diabetes, I had finished reading your book about when you got diabetes ... so, I immediately switched to a low-carb diet. Four weeks later, I was back at the clinic to try out blood sugar meters. She picked one, showed me how it worked, stuck me in the finger and the device began to beep. This was after lunch, and the meter displayed 5.5 ... the nurse picked it up, shook it and glared skeptically at it, muttering that it must be broken. Let's try another one, she said. The next sample showed 5.3. Then she rushed out of the room to consult with my doctor.

Anyway, they gave me a meter to take home, with a lot of instructions and dietary advice that I honestly did not follow. My blood sugar has been stable since then, varying between 5.0 and 7.2; it's generally between 5.5 and 6.5. I haven't taken any medication or insulin.

Now I feel just great. Sticking to my low-carb diet has never been a problem. I used to eat all the time, any time, and I was chronically hungry ... now I only eat twice a day. I have a few nuts and some cheese as a snack during the day when I feel like it.

I eat a hearty breakfast consisting of an omelette, usually stuffed with mushrooms and ham and lots of grated cheese (after six months I got tired of bacon and eggs). During the *day I usually don't eat anything, I just drink lots of cafe latte and water. I also always include yogurt for breakfast. Dinnertime is at about 7 to 8 p.m. I'm tall and stout (200 cm, 133 kg at my heaviest).*

Now I've lost 13 kg. I guess I should lose more weight, but I'm not worried. I'll get there.

Here's some info about my previous symptoms: Diabetes, ulcers, chronic hunger, stomach pains, heart palpitations, allergic symptoms – much improved, migraine, stronger immune system. Dizziness. Less need for sleep, bedtime 3:00 and up at 8:30. I've taken Losec for the past five years as well as Seloken (ulcers and heart palpitations). I've now stopped taking all of these medications!

My wife even says my penis has grown larger, but I don't think so. It probably just looks bigger because my belly doesn't hang down as far, if you know what I mean …

Anders, age 43

Jeanette

This story is from the mother of a child diagnosed with type 1 diabetes:

My son, who is 17, contracted diabetes in April this year. We were in hospital for a week and he was receiving 102 units of *insulin each day at the time we were sent home. The hospital served "regular" food :(*

When we got home, we combed the Internet for information, and found a variety of sites, including your website. We realised that carbs are out … We gradually reduced insulin dosage while reducing the carbs.

A month later, he was insulin-free!!!!! He only takes insulin when he feels like eating a sandwich or is tempted by some potato chips (once a week or so). His long-term blood Sugar (Hba1C) fell from 14.5 to 5.9 in just over four months. All the other test values and his weight are good. During our last visit, the doctor said that Isaac shouldn't make any changes.

It's been seven months now since his diabetes diagnosis, so we realise that he might need some maintenance level insulin later on. But imagine the amount of insulin that he has not had to inject!!!!! And this simply by skipping the foods he doesn't tolerate … it's actually quite obvious. Everyone at the hospital said he should eat whatever he wants and keep using insulin!!

Today, 4 of 8 family members are on THE SCANDINAVIAN DIET … and we feel just greeeaat :)

All the best, Jeanette

Egil

I'd also like to tell you about my contact with Egil from Norway. He's a type 2 diabetic, and began to follow the advice in my book after reading the Norwegian edition. Blood sugar levels improved quite soon after cutting down on carbohydrates. Egil wasn't the least bit afraid of pricking his finger to measure blood sugar, and he made quite detailed measurements. The upper curve shows his blood sugar levels on a conventional diet, the one recommended to diabetics. The lower curve shows blood sugar levels on THE SCANDINAVIAN DIET. Blood sugar values peaked at 20 on the high carb and low-fat diet, whereas on THE SCANDINAVIAN DIET, they did not go over 10.

Both curves show results without medication or insulin. Egil took insulin (12 units) and Metformin before starting with THE SCANDINAVIAN DIET. His blood sugar level was usually around 10 in the morning, and about 14 or 15 after meals, peaking at 23. The curve shows how proper food can be better than insulin.

Egil tells me that his blood sugar level is stable today at between 4.7 and 5.3. It doesn't exceed 8 – 9 two hours after meals. He's 6 feet (179 cm) tall and weighs 160lbs (73 kg). His blood sugar values are good in spite of taking medication for other diseases that slightly elevate blood sugar.

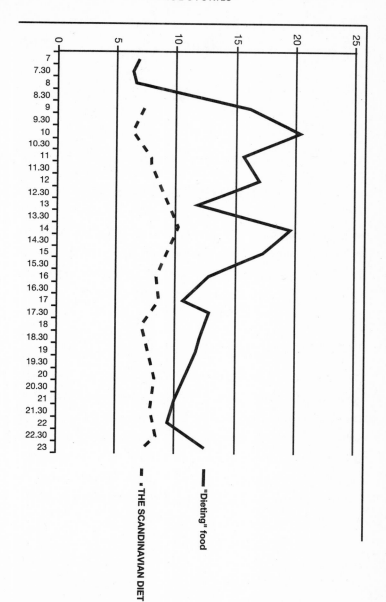

Why is there no progress in diabetes treatment?

Some of the advocates of today's dietary advice use defensive techniques that one wouldn't think were permitted in an open society. Here are some examples of what happens when one tries to question the established dogma.

The food industry supplies us with "facts"

On November 16, 2008, the Swedish investigative journalism program "Cold Facts" aired an episode about modern dietary advice. Professor Nils Georg Asp, chairman of the Swedish Nutrition Foundation, was one of the interviewees. Asp is known for his liberal views about sugar, even for diabetics. Here is an excerpt of the interview regarding the brochure "Good food for all – a diet for people with diabetes and heart disease":

Nils-Georg Asp:
I helped produce this brochure about 20 years ago ...

Reporter Johan Åsard:
Do you think that it's still valid?

Asp:
Yes, basically, I do. Hmm.

Reporter:
It suggests a lot of carbohydrates?

Asp:
Uh, yes …

Reporter:
*Carbohydrates elevate blood sugar, which requires more insulin.
Is this good for a diabetic?*

Asp:
Hm … uhh … if you eat good carbohydrates…

Reporter:
*So, wouldn't it be smart to eat food that doesn't elevate blood
sugar?*

Asp:
*Eh … certainly … it might appear so … but with proper treat-
ment … uh … a … a person with diabetes can metabolise these
carbohydrates.*

Reporter:
And by proper treatment you mean insulin and medication?

Asp:
Eh… yes, if required.

Danisco Sugar is one of the members of the Swedish Nutrition Foundation, and of course they don't want sugar to be presented as dangerous for diabetics. Nils Georg Asp is performing his duties well by telling us that sugar isn't a problem for a diabetic. Just take your medicine if you need it. And you will need it.

As long as there are individuals with this attitude about the health benefits of sugar and starch for diabetics, and especially if they're allowed to produce brochures for diabetics – they'll be preventing diabetics from living a symptom-free life without medication. I really hope that future generations will not have to read brochures like "Good food for all". Nobody deserves a brochure that functions as advertising for food producers who make products that make diabetics even sicker. I'll leave it up to the reader to form an opinion about a person who, contrary to his own better knowledge, produces brochures with counterproductive dietary advice. My own opinions about this are not fit to print.

Manipulating the facts

When the Swedish Royal Academy of Science held a symposium* on obesity and diabetes on November 20, 2008, the first speaker, Ellen Blaak, spoke about the so-called "Israel Study", the most extensive weight loss study to date, which compared low-fat diets to Mediterranean diets and low-carb diets. The study was well-designed and conducted, and lasted for two years. It showed us that those who ate the least amount of carbohydrates lost the most weight. In contrast to the low-fat group and Mediterranean diet group, the low-carb group had no caloric restrictions, and could eat as much as they wanted. The only rule was to restrict the amount of carbohydrates. They could, in other words, eat *ad libitum*, meaning they could eat as much as they wanted. The speaker did not, however, report these astounding facts. Isn't it quite peculiar that those who could eat as much as they wanted lost the most weight?

Instead, the following conclusion was presented on one slide: "Under ad libitum conditions, low fat diets result in a higher body weight loss."

This conclusion is exactly the opposite of what the results of the Israeli study demonstrated. The speaker based these statements on a meta-study (study of a study) done by the Danish diet professor Arne Astrup. Unfortunately, he did not

---

* At the time of writing, the symposium is available at
  mms://wmedia.it.su.se/kv/kva081120.wmv

elaborate on these contradictory results, but simply ignored the Israeli study.

In the summary, Astrup's meta-analysis forms the basis of the conclusion that, if allowed to eat as much as desired, maximum weight loss was achieved by a low-fat diet.

It would seem reasonable that at least one person in the well-informed audience would have reacted. Especially because the Israeli study was widely quoted when it was published in the summer of 2008. Seemingly, no one in the audience reacted to the distortion of facts during the presentation. The speaker was a professor, so whatever he was saying must be reasonable?

Was there an intentional cover-up of the results of the Israeli study? I can only conclude that, just as in love and war, all is fair in the diet debate. This does look like a clumsy repetition of Ancel Keys' experimental fraud of the 1950's.* For some reason, no effort was spared to create a negative image of the low-carb diet. What are we afraid of?

One explanation for this peculiar behaviour could be that the speaker was associated with ILSI, International Life Science Institute, a lobby organisation that is financed by companies such as Danisco Sugar, the Danish sugar giant that also financed Arne Astrup's research. It would be disastrous if it became widely known that more effective weight loss could be achieved by a low-carb diet.

If the speaker were better-versed in his subject, he might

* More information in "Fear of Fat", Optimal Publishing.

have been able to successfully criticise the Israeli study. Perhaps it was his connection to ILSI that prevented him from correctly and properly presenting the results of the Israeli study.

In the meantime, we'll have to make do with the old and politically correct "truths", in line with what the food industry wants us to think.

Experts, bought and paid for

It's more common than you might imagine that diet experts associated with government health authorities are actually working for the food and pharmaceutical industries. Biting the hand that feeds you is not something you readily do, and as a result, we can see that advice about our diet is resistant to change. The book *Ideologin och pengarna bakom kostråden* (Ideology and Money Behind Dietary Advice, Pagina Publishers 2007) further examines this subject. It's also more common than you would imagine that these shady connections are not openly admitted, except as a result of direct confrontation.

The phenomenon of "Acting Professor" seems quite strange, as a corporation can simply buy a title for a handpicked expert and then let them act as if they were a professor. The Professor title implies true expertise, but this need not always be the case. Basically anyone can be bestowed with such a title, and then act in the name of their employer while the general public believes that they are actually an academic professor.

Quite a lot of publicity will be needed before any changes

can be made. Every time results are published from studies which demonstrate that today's dietary advice is not correct, we hear that this is a "single result" (which, of course, it is), and that we can't make any changes on the basis of a single result. So the question is, how many individual studies need to be done before we will take note? Or maybe the guardians of the status quo need to leave the arena and allow room for a new generation, one that has learned to think differently? Unfortunately, it looks like we have a long wait before the retirement of the so-called experts who have been trained by today's establishment.

A common objection to even thinking about changing today's dietary advice is: "If people just listened to the advice, everything would be much better." There are increasing numbers of studies showing that, even if one dutifully follows today's dietary advice, it's still a less-healthy diet compared to a low carbohydrate diet, regardless of how it is measured. This objection doesn't stand up to scrutiny.

One might even begin to think that this business of "which foods are good for you?" has little to do with science. A wise man once told me that medicine is the least intellectual of scientific disciplines. The more I learn about how it works, the more I'm inclined to agree. Basically, what is supposed to be good for you is all about the money. Food producers are allowed to participate in dietary advice decisions. We're talking about multinational corporations such as Coca-Cola and the other food giants. Obviously, food producers want to produce products cheaply and sell them at a high price. Corporations must generate profits, and they have found that the easiest way to do that is to sell diluted products on the grounds that they are healthy, but for at least the same price as the "real deal".

Dubious studies

We would like to believe that medical research can be trusted. But there's also a difference between the actual conclusions of a study and how they are published.

The food industry has a vested interest in presenting the preferred results of the studies that they have paid for. There's more than one way to get that done. One can exaggerate the significance of positive results, or one can simply choose to not publish results from studies that do not benefit the company. It's been said that positive studies are published three times more often than negative studies. One can also manipulate the data. Of course, this is nothing new or surprising. I found the following quote in the Swedish medical press* *"Chief editor of the JAMA (Journal of the American Medical Association) Catherine DeAngelis, for example, writes in her April editorial that the medical and research professions have been swamped with lobbyists from pharmaceutical companies, and it's time to stop it now. Her point is that manipulation and misrepresentation of research results by profiting corporations is only possible because investigators, editors, reviewers and authorities actively cooperate with the corporations. She then*

---

* *Läkartidningen* 2008-10-21: "Kan man lita på kliniska studier", Fredrik Hedlund, freelance journalist.

proposes an eleven-point program to minimise the possibility for corporations to manipulate medical research.

Marcia Angell, ex-editor of the New England Journal of Medicine, said that, after 20 years at her post, research reports financed by corporations on the efficacy and side effects of drugs could no longer be trusted. She also comments in JAMA that the only thing one can be sure of is that positive effects of drugs reported in corporate-financed studies are in all likelihood significantly lower than those that are presented in the report.

Because virtually all of the supplemental training for physicians comes from the pharmaceutical industry, it's not hard to imagine that the industry succeeds in achieving their goals. How can a doctor know what the results of a study really mean if they are adjusted to satisfy special interest groups?

One study* examined how food industry-financed research was reported. It was shown that studies financed by companies with economic interests in the product were between four and eight times more likely to report a positive result, as compared to studies not financed by corporate interests. The study concluded that corporate sponsors might only sponsor research if they are sure about a positive result. Or, one can formulate hypotheses that agree with the sponsor's interests. Conversely, results that are in conflict with the sponsor's interests might not be published. In addition, review articles might only include studies that benefit the sponsor.

* Lesser LI, Ebbeling CB, Goozner M, Wypij D, Ludwig DS (2007) Relationship between Funding Source and Conclusion among Nutrition-Related Scientific Articles. PLoS Med 4(1): e5. Doi:10. 1371/journal.pmed.0040005

One of the solutions proposed in the study to fix this problem would be to increase the level of government funding.

Profit motives in the pharmaceutical industry

Drug companies are just like any other company. Shareholders are naturally interested in receiving dividends. This applies to all for-profit corporations, and is not in the least unusual. Companies that cannot generate a profit are simply not going to survive. On the other hand, pharmaceutical companies are subject to extraordinary conflicts of interest.

From the perspective of a pharmaceutical company and its management, it's obvious that the more people who have illnesses that require medication, the better. The perfect citizen will live a long, unhealthy life and will use as much medicine as possible. The fact that more than 5% of the populace suffers from diabetes represents quite a cash cow. The upper limits for the diagnosis of high blood pressure, diabetes and high cholesterol have declined in recent years, resulting in greater numbers of people on prescription medication.

Cholesterol medications (statins) are extremely profitable, and research to discover and patent new medications is constantly ongoing. The definition of "high" cholesterol is continually being lowered, resulting in an increased numbers of prescriptions. Drugs are being prescribed to combat a natural substance which is found in mother's milk and is required for cell membrane and brain function, and the production of sex hormones. It also protects us against infections. New drugs are constantly being introduced even when they do not reduce mortality rates. Statins, on the contrary, have many side effects. For example, they interfere with production of coenzyme Q10, which the heart and other muscles need to function properly.

We can conclude that pharmaceutical companies are just as cold and calculating as any other corporation. My own experience tells me that pharmaceutical companies are not interested in seeing diabetics become healthy on their own, which is not surprising.

I would have no objection if doctors acted on their experience and conscience, treating diabetic patients to help them become symptom-free, but this is not the case. Doctors do not want to take risks, and it's safer just to stay within the mainstream. Despite the fact that diabetics will surely get worse as a result of treatment.

Fear of reprimands

Physician Annika Dahlqvist displayed considerable courage when she recommended THE SCANDINAVIAN DIET to diabetics and obese patients, and she was subsequently reported to the authorities by dieticians for not adhering to science and proven experience. Her license to practice medicine hung in the balance. Fortunately, the National Board of Health and Welfare came to the conclusion that a low-carbohydrate diet was in agreement with science and proven experience for treatment of diabetes and obesity. One may be inclined to sympathise with doctors who dare not treat their patients and help them become symptom-free, if this treatment exposes them to the risk of being reported to the authorities by their colleagues.

Chief physician Jörgen Vesti-Nielsen in Karlshamn was in charge of the Karlshamns study, which I have previously described in this book. In that study, one group of patients ate according to the plate model, while the other group ate fewer carbohydrates and more fat. He was also reported – by the chairman of the Swedish Dietitians Association. Vesti-Nielsen was eventually exonerated by the National Board of Health and Welfare. One can conclude that doctors who are seriously interested in trying to help their patients put themselves at risk.

The importance of profit

The drug industry prefers the status quo. That way diabetics need lots of medicine, which is good for business. Pharmaceutical companies have the resources to organise seminars for doctors, much more so than the public sector has. This means that those doctors are presented "truths" prepared by the drug companies. So in reality, diabetics would be wise to remember that their health will not improve by following the advice of drug companies or the doctors trained by those companies. According to some calculations, doing the exact opposite of what we are told to do by the most renowned diet professor in Sweden will result in a net health benefit to both society and the individual.

People who suffer from diabetes and/or obesity should be

very wary and sceptical of "official" dietary advice. There's a reason for this advice, and the reason has little to do with the patient's best interests.

Economic dependence

I've spent some time leafing through two years of back issues of the magazine "Diabetes", published by the Swedish Diabetes Association. On average, 22% of the magazine consists of advertisements. One of the most popular advertisements is for blood sugar meters. The advertising revenue generated in each issue is somewhere between 30 000 and 60 000 US dollars. If the magazine is to survive, these advertisements must be sold. Here we have a conundrum. What freedom does the editorial staff of the magazine have to critically examine the products made and sold by the advertisers who support them? We often say that if you can't beat them, join them. What would motivate the magazine to publish articles with information that might free diabetics from the need for devices and medication?

Fear of rocking the boat

It seems that a lot of toes will stepped on if one tries to enlighten diabetics about the paths to improved health without medicine. A few years ago, I volunteered to speak at a diabetes association meeting in Sweden about my experience in rejecting the conventional dietary wisdom. By way of a third party, I came across a flyer that had subsequently been printed. This flyer had been mailed to each and every diabetes association in Sweden. Here is what it said:

"Hello everyone!
This is to enquire whether you too have received mail from this man. We can under no circumstances endorse this diet. It has nothing to do with science and proven experience. We hope that you will act as we did – say NO!
Regards, Anita!"

I should add that the Swedish National Board of Health and Welfare concurs that THE SCANDINAVIAN DIET is in agreement with science and proven experience.

Medication: The only solution?

Not every diabetes association that received this flyer acted on their recommendation, and I have made presentations for various diabetes associations in Sweden. In one case, I later heard that a local pharmacy had significantly reduced their sales of insulin. The local chairman of the diabetes association was taken to task for this, as it was concluded that his invitation along with my presentation, were responsible for people not buying as much insulin as they had previously. This was regarded as dangerous. Obviously, not taking needed insulin can be hazardous, but imagine if we could at least consider the possibility that diabetics might not need to take as much insulin? What if they just became healthier? This thought does not seem to cross the minds of my critics.

Self-interest

Let's not forget that "caring" for the patients can also disguise a degree of self-interest. Taking care of diabetics can be profitable. I received a copy of a letter sent by a diabetes nurse to a number of diabetes associations, as well as to Bayer, Medi-Sense, Novo Nordisk and Roche Diagnostics. In her letter, she complained that some diabetes associations had been in touch with manufacturers of blood-sugar meters and test strips in order to offer these items to new members, either free or at a low cost. She wrote that soliciting new memberships by offering these meters was in itself wrong. Membership should be based on personal interest, and not as a way to get a free blood-sugar meter. In her opinion, patients needed information and training to use these meters, and for this reason, providing them for free was wrong.

Generally, patients pay a certain sum to the diabetes nurse for the meter. I've heard that this payment is seen as an unofficial bonus to the nurse. In view of this, it's easy to understand the resentment when diabetes associations provide the meters for free.

Fear of information reaching diabetics

After I finished the manuscript for my first book, *Fettskrämd* (Fear of Fat), I contacted the Swedish website "Allt om diabetes" (Everything about Diabetes) to see if they were interested in reviewing my book. This website is about managing diabetes, and I thought it would be a perfect match for them to review my book, because it was about how to become a symptom-free diabetic. Things seemed promising at first. I sent them a PDF copy of the manuscript, and they promised to get back to me in a couple of weeks when the editorial staff returned. The weeks passed, and I waited in vain for a reply. I tried to get in touch with them again, but to no avail. This aroused my suspicion. At first, I thought that perhaps my book was so terrible that they didn't want to review it. This seemed strange, however, because Lars Werkö, one of Sweden's most respected professors of medicine, had written a foreword praising the book.

At that point I decided to find out who was running this website. Maybe that would provide an explanation? It turned out that the web site was owned by Novo Nordisk, a company that produces, among other things, insulin and injection equipment. I now understand that they would be foolish to write about my book. I'm still waiting for an explanation for their total silence. If diabetics would start to follow the advice in my book, insulin sales would drop significantly. As a matter of fact, every diabetic I know who has switched from so-called "healthy" food to eating according to THE SCANDINAVIAN DIET, has also experienced improved health. I have yet to hear of an exception.

I've also informed the Merck-owned website www.diabetesinfo.se about this book, and received the following negative reply with no further explanation:

"Hello,
Thank you for your e-mail. Unfortunately, it is impossible
for us to write about your book.
  Good luck!"

Apparently, these websites have no genuine interest in the health of diabetics, but rather in their own profit margin. They could have informed their readership about my book, how bad it was and how they should avoid it, but they chose silence instead. They didn't want to risk generating any debate, because they had nothing to gain. That explains the silence.

Ignorant and dangerous dieticians

So-called "experts" cannot be trusted. An "expert" may have vested economic interests that cast a shadow on their opinions. Even after years of training, there's no guarantee that an "expert" hasn't got it wrong anyway. The risk of losing face often prevents people from changing their opinions, so they cling harder to those opinions instead. Eva Kullenberg, registered dietician, is a good example. In her blog she enthusiastically encourages us to eat more berries, fruit and vegetables. At the request of the reader, she expounds on the role of insulin. She writes: *"Insulin is a protein essential to life, necessary to convert what we eat into blood sugar"* (!)

If an insulin-dependent diabetic would read this and take it at face value, he or she wouldn't dare take an insulin injection, because according to Eva Kullenberg, insulin *elevates* blood sugar. According to her, insulin transforms food into sugar in the blood. Despite repeated requests for an explanation or reference, she has not answered. So, at the time of writing, she still maintains that insulin transforms food into blood sugar. The truth is that insulin lowers blood sugar by making it accessible to the cells in the body. This is dangerous and ignorant behaviour from a registered dietician, someone we should be able to trust.

Flight from accountability

When doing something on your own, you're 100% responsible. If you share the responsibility with others, you feel maybe 1% responsible. The "follow-the-leader" mentality kicks in. I recently read an article about dietary advice in the Swedish medical journal *Läkartidningen*. One of the authors of the article was Elisabet Rothenberg, chairman of the National Association of Dieticians. Here is what I wrote in an e-mail to Rothenberg:

Hello,

In Läkartidningen *there is a statement written by Claude Marcus et al, including yourself, to The National Board of Health and Welfare in reply to your original article.*

Regarding a low carbohydrate diet, you wrote that it is **"inappropriate and in some cases directly harmful"***. The National Board of Health and Welfare did not substantiate this claim, nor did Stephan Rössner, who claimed that*

such a diet is not harmful, only boring. What scientific basis
do you have for this statement?

    Best regards,
    Lars-Erik Litsfeldt

I received the following reply:

Lars-Erik,

In a free country one may entertain whatever opinion one
desires. It's a good thing, however, if it's supported by
good reasoning. I have nothing to say in addition to what
I have already stated,

    Best regards,
    Elisabet Rothenberg
    Chief nutritionist, MD
    Department of Clinical Nutrition,
    Sahlgrenska University Hospital

In this case, Dr. Rothenberg has no basis for her statement.
Had there been, she would certainly have pointed it out to me.
Instead, I was told that in a free country, one is entitled to
one's opinion. And I thought that *Läkartidningen* didn't print
statements based on casual opinions. Are there really no
requirements on scientific evidence? How would people who
are less well-versed in the peculiarities of academia interpret
this? Is modern dietary advice simply a matter of opinion,
with no scientific basis?

One amusing detail is that, as a reference in support of the
claim that dietary fibre, fruit and vegetables had a positive

effect on blood fats, authors Claude Marcus, Göran Hallmans, Gunnar Johansson, Elisabet Rothenberg and Stephan Rössner cited a publication about the presence of Listeria bacteria in sausage meat.* None of the authors noticed this glaring error. Do any of them check their references? And why didn't *Läkartidningen* notice anything? What will they print next? Research scientist Johan Hedbrant wrote the following comments in a letter to the same journal:

> *That the "sausage meat" reference was included "by mistake" is not a surprising excuse. :-)*
>
> *I'd also like to see an explanation of how four professors, the National Association of Dieticians, the ten or so research scientists and nutritional experts who contributed to this article, as well as the editors of the Journal did not discover this, in light of the fact that the debate was in part focused on the lack of scientific foundation for dietary recommendations.*
>
> *http://www.lakartidningen.se/engine.php?articleId=9461*
> *Who bears the actual responsibility for the accuracy of scientific publications?*
> *Johan Hedbrant*
> *Research investigator, University of Linköping*

This really hit the nail on the head.

* Frankfurtersausage.

Consensus

It also seems that, when people are in agreement, it's a sign that what they agree on is true. We hear this quite often. *"There is a consensus regarding this issue"* or *"This is in no way controversial, all the leading experts are in agreement"*. I think we should return to Johan Hedbrant and his comments regarding this thing we call consensus:

"Science is driven by controversy, not by agreement. It is within this sort of intellectual exchange that science develops.

Science is basically an open forum, where "everyone" is able to examine the foundations of various theories. It's fascinating that this debate seems to always end with each camp slinging references at one another and sticking to their interpretation. "Everyone" does not have the same possibility to search the original literature and evaluate various interpretations.

Who "everyone" trusts becomes a question of credibility, and instead of examining detailed evidence, trust is based on the authority of the source, as well as their capacity to describe reality in terms that "everyone" recognises.

How can we further advance science, beyond this barrier?"

We should be thankful for those individuals who have the courage to stand up to this herd of experts who all "know" that they are right. Copernicus suspected that the Earth orbits the Sun, not the other way around. The consensus in those days was that the Sun revolves around the Earth. If we had continued to agree with each other, we would still believe that, and anyone who maintained otherwise would be labelled a freak and be ostracised.

We can nevertheless be thankful that consensus decisions are not made automatically. During the Swedish Heart and Lung Association symposium in October 2008, Professor Claude Marcus pleaded for a consensus regarding the risks of saturated fats. This consensus was not reached because the attending scientists, quite correctly, did not think there was sufficient scientific evidence for such a decision.

In the spring of 2007, associate professor Uffe Ravnskov contacted Ronald Krauss, ex-chairman of the Nutrition Committee in the USA. Krauss had discovered that the more tiny LDL particles present in the blood, the higher the risk of a fatal heart attack. Krauss had also succeeded in demonstrating that a high intake of saturated fat resulted in a decrease in the number of these tiny dense particles. We have otherwise been trained to fear saturated fats, which makes this quite an intriguing discovery. Uffe Ravnskov asked Krauss why mainstream opinion maintained that saturated fats were unhealthy. Ronald Krauss replied: "*You see, if the members of the committee disagree, we take a vote, and the majority of the committee members determine the committee's opinion.*"

In other words, they can vote to decide what is good and what is bad for the rest of us. One might easily think that this story is from the Middle Ages, but that's unfortunately not so. But this is what happens when scientific evidence is inconclusive.

The Swedish National Food Administration often defers to expert committees in unanimous agreement about, among other things, the dangers of saturated fat. Well, we now know what that can mean.

Expert committees are only needed when the evidence is controversial. In order to make a decision, we leave it to the experts to agree on what is probably true. The general public often confuses these decisions with proven scientific facts.

In the book *Ideologin, pengarna och kostråden* (Ideology, Money and Dietary Advice) which I co-authored with Per Wikholm, we clearly outlined the relationships between members of the expert committees and their industrial interests. Anyone on the payroll of an industrial bakery is likely to claim that whole-wheat bread is good for you. This conflict of interest was not always reported. There has been a casual attitude towards these "declarations of disqualification", and stricter regulations have recently been adopted, only after publication of the book. We now have examples of experts who have suddenly rescued themselves from these expert groups. When their bias was questioned, some of these experts threatened to "go on strike", which is somewhat touching. They want to continue their activities undisturbed, and don't appreciate being questioned.

Connections to the food industry can obviously bias the results of an expert committee. Lars-Erik Holm, the recently appointed chief of the National Board of Health and Welfare, showed some gumption by firing Bengt Vessby and Nils Georg Asp from the committee to develop new dietary advice for diabetics. Bengt Vessby is on the payroll of e.g. Dansukker, and Nils Georg Asp is the CEO of Swedish Nutrition Foundation, a food industry lobbying organisation. Asp is also a member of ILSI, a global lobby organization headquartered in the USA. The European Union is funding ILSI with €13,000,000 for the task of creating new dietary guidelines for European Union member states. ILSI Europe members:

Ajinomoto
Akzo Nobel Functional Chemicals
Barilla G. & R. F.lli
BASF
Bayer CropScience Bioscience
Beverages Partners Worldwide
bioMérieux Industry
Campina
Cereal Partners Worldwide
Cerestar
Coca-Cola European Union Group
Cognis
Colloïdes Naturels International
Danisco Sweeteners
Dow Europe
DSM
Firmenich
Friesland Foods
Givaudan
GlaxoSmithKline
Groupe Danone

H.J. Heinz
Kellogg Company
Kraft Foods International
L'Oréal
Masterfoods
McDonald's Europe
McNeil Nutritionals
Mead Johnson Nutritionals
Monsanto Europe
National Starch Food Innovation
Nestlé
PepsiCo International
Procter & Gamble
Raffinerie Tirlemontoise — ORAFTI
Raisio Group
Red Bull
RHM Technology
Roquette Frères
Royal Ahold
Royal Cosun
Royal Numico
Seven Seas
Südzucker
Swiss Quality Testing Services
Tate & Lyle Specialty Sweeteners
Tetra Pak Research
The Valspar Corporation
Unilever
Valio

WILD Flavours/Ingredients
Yakult

I'm reluctant to even contemplate the kind of dietary advice we can expect from ILSI-members such as Coca-Cola and Kellogg's. Monsanto, another member, is well-known for products such as genetically-modified crops and the defoliant Agent Orange, which was used to strip the jungles of Vietnam. I'm not quite comfortable knowing that these companies have influence over what we are recommended to eat.

Obfuscation/convolution

One way to avoid important but undesired subjects is to begin talking about other, completely irrelevant things. Not long ago, I observed a seminar on the Internet regarding the existence of health hazards due to saturated fat. This question certainly deserves to be examined. An English counterpart to the Head of the National Food Administration continually changed the subject to how successful they were at reducing salt intake. Obfuscating the topic is a popular trick.

Disparaging salt intake is politically quite correct. In addition, very few people would care to make an issue of that.

If we eat too much salt, we become thirsty, we drink and excrete the salt in our urine – end of story. Problems with too little salt are much more common – as we cannot store salt in our bodies for future use. Without enough salt, we experience circulatory problems that can even lead to death.

The salt debate is about a gram here and a gram there.

Convolution is a way to shift the focus to unimportant or irrelevant information that no-one cares about. Saying something true but irrelevant to an "information consumer" will lead them to think that what one says about the "other" topic is also true; a nifty trick in a debate.

Lack of logic

It's strange that, even today, a major portion of the dietary intake recommended to diabetics consists precisely of that which makes them sick. We don't ask people with peanut allergies to carry inhalers in order to continue eating peanuts. Instead, we recommend avoiding peanuts. This does not seem to apply to diabetics. Diabetics should eat things they cannot tolerate, and then counteract the ill effects with medication.

Conclusion

Type 1 and type 2 diabetes are serious conditions that you should seek to prevent now. There's so much to be gained. For type 2 diabetics, the advantages are obvious. Type 1 diabetics will benefit from cutting down on carbohydrates and replacing them with natural fat. If you want to avoid vision problems, infected feet or amputation, kidney problems etc., you must take care of your body. It's not as bad as it sounds. All you need to do is eat those foods to which your body is adapted. Sugar and starch, as we know, promote dental cavities. We can hardly say we're adapted to things that cause problems when we put them in our mouths.

The alternative foods are not bad at all. Scrambled eggs and bacon with a pat of butter can be your breakfast. You can eat meat and fish, no matter what colour. Cover it with some delicious rich sauce. Use full-fat sour cream. Professional chefs love to use real butter, cream and salt in their dishes, and now you can use the same ingredients. Without a bad conscience!

You'll run into people who disagree with you, and you'll read about studies that conflict with what you've learned from this book. Keep an open mind and absorb the information. You might learn something. Unfortunately, there is a lot of dubious information out there. It's often difficult to recognise. One tried-and-true method is to follow the money. Who paid for the study? You can't imagine what interests lie behind medical studies. They could be manufacturers of breakfast flakes, sugar, pasta or sugary beverages. Do the results of the studies seem to agree with what the sponsor might want? If so, you should examine the study carefully and make sure that it was conducted properly, and also that it was published in an objective manner.

I cannot, for the life of me, understand how one can maintain that a diabetic should eat sugar. It shouldn't be difficult to realise that people who become ill from sugar and starch shouldn't eat it. Despite all that, we continue on the same old path, stay wary of fat and tell ourselves to eat those so-called slow carbs. Even slow carbohydrates elevate blood sugar, it's just that the elevation continues for a longer time. This causes even more harm to our body. I don't envy those who stubbornly insist that diabetics should eat starch. One day we'll rediscover that sugar and starch is bad for diabetics. How many feet will be amputated before our diet advice reflects the truth?

Too many people have suffered unnecessarily in recent decades, while starch has had free rein over the diabetic's diet. "Deferred complications" were regarded as natural and to be expected. Many premature deaths from coronary disease due to inflammation have been caused by high insulin levels in combination with high blood sugar levels.

Over 2400 years ago, in ancient Greece, public servant and orator Lysias mentioned in passing: *"You have heard, you have seen, you have suffered. It is in your grasp. Give your verdict."*

I can only agree.

Recipes

Egg dishes

Eggs are nature's own smart food.

They contain plenty of the nutrients we need for our health and well-being, such as vitamins A, B2 (riboflavin), D and E, calcium, selenium and zinc.

Eggs also contain lots of protein (egg white) and fat (egg yolk).

Check the quality! Eggs from free-range hens are much more nutritious than the cheap eggs from hens raised in egg factories. Organic eggs are better and tastier!

Poached eggs

Boil some water in a wide saucepan with a pinch of salt and a few drops of vinegar. Reduce the heat to a simmer.

Crack an egg onto a plate with a little water.

Slowly slide the egg from the plate into the centre of the saucepan. When the egg white becomes firm, it's ready to serve. If you want a visible yolk, use less water in the saucepan. For an elegant touch, remove the ragged edges using an inverted water glass as a cutter.

Tasty garnishes might include a dab of natural or flavoured sour cream or caviar sauce.

Scrambled eggs

Scrambled eggs provide for endless variations and can be served with bacon, ham, broccoli, smoked fish etc.

Scrambled eggs for one

2 whole eggs, 4 tablespoons cream or crème fraiche, salt, ground nutmeg

Melt a generous dab of butter in a pan.

Crack the eggs into the pan. Stir, remove from the heat occasionally and continue stirring. When the eggs start to become firm, add cream and continue stirring. Add a bit of salt. Remove from the heat before it looks ready, because it will continue to harden. Scrambled eggs are tastier when served somewhat creamy.

A hint of nutmeg adds flavour to all egg dishes.

Omelettes

Inspiration for the two following omelette recipes comes from a cookbook printed in 1902. That's before we were scared of fat.

With a fork, whisk three eggs, some melted butter and a couple of tablespoons of semi skimmed milk.

Heat the mixture on a greased iron or frying pan. When it

begins to set, spread your chosen stuffing on half of the omelette. Prepare the stuffing using fish, crayfish tails, creamed spinach or whatever suits your taste. When the omelette is golden brown on the underside, use a spatula to fold it over on the half covered with stuffing.

You can also use this recipe for pancakes; serve as an appetiser with caviar or other roe, crème fraiche and a bit of chopped dill and onion.

For dessert, garnish the pancakes with berries and whipped cream.

THE SCANDINAVIAN DIET-type stuffing is easily prepared using crème fraiche and/or cream cheese. Just mix, for example, chopped spinach leaves with crème fraiche or cream cheese. If you have diabetes, try to avoid flour, which is high in carbohydrates.

Cheese omelette

This recipe is also more than one hundred years old!

Use a fork to combine the eggs and butter until the mixture becomes a bit frothy. Do not whisk.

Add 50 g (1.75 oz) of butter to a frying pan. Pour the egg mixture into the pan, stirring carefully until it begins to solidify. Do not whisk! Shake the pan gently now and again. Distribute the cheese and fold the omelette in half.

Slide carefully onto a plate.

The real-life Swedish chef, Tore Wretman, also a world-renowned omelette expert, was always careful to remove it from the heat before it solidified completely. I generally follow his advice.

Fluffy microwaved eggs

Making scrambled eggs in the microwave is simple, and is especially suited for one or two people.

Mix the ingredients in a microwave-safe bowl (i.e. not metal). Plastic and porcelain work well. Cook at full heat for 30 to 60 seconds, depending on the oven.

Remove from the microwave and stir the warm mixture. Return it to the oven and cook at full heat for 30 to 60 seconds, depending on the oven. Remove from the microwave and stir the warm mixture. If the eggs are still runny, heat them again for a few seconds. When the mixture has congealed to a soft and fluffy texture, the dish is ready to serve!

As always, add spice and garnish according to your taste. A little nutmeg is delicious.

Fish dishes

Fish in its various forms is a perfect health food. We've all heard that "eating fish makes you smart."

A fish diet also keeps you healthy and alert as it contains plenty of the healthy omega-3 fatty acids.

If you never eat fish, you may require a dietary supplement in the form of omega-3 capsules. Fish also contain plenty of healthy protein, which you need to fill that perfect body.

Crispy salmon

Preheat the oven to 225°C.

Peel the garlic and onions and cut the onions into wedges. Remove the stalks from the parsley and basil.

Chop the onions, herbs and nuts in a blender until the mixture is smooth and green. Add salt, pepper and fruit juice.

Place the salmon on a sheet of baking paper in an oven-safe deep dish. Spread the nut mixture over the fish. Bake in the oven for 15 to 20 minutes, until the salmon is cooked and the topping has a nice colour. Frozen salmon may require an additional five minutes in the oven.

Tasty side dishes include vegetables sautéed in butter, ratatouille and wok-fried vegetables (see page 181).

Grilled salmon with pesto

Ingredients, serves 4: 4 fillets of salmon (150 g (5.3 oz) each), 100 g (3.5 oz) hazelnuts, 1 garlic clove, 3 shallots, (or yellow onion), 1 sprig parsley, 1 sprig basil, juice of ½ lemon or 1 lime, salt and pepper.

Combine all the ingredients for the pesto in a blender.

Melt the butter in a frying pan. When the butter stops sizzling, fry the fish with the skin facing downward. Salt and pepper to taste.

Cover the fish with a saucepan lid or plate and let it finish cooking at low heat. Don't overcook.

Serve the pesto with the fish as it is or heat it up in a thick-bottomed saucepan.

Serve with a salad.

Fillet of salmon with bacon

Ingredients, serves 4: 4 salmon fillets, about 140 g (5 oz) each, 1 package bacon, butter for the pan.

Preheat the oven to 225°C.

Wrap the bacon around the fish and place the fillets in a buttered oven dish.

Cook for 15–20 minutes; deep-frozen fillets require about 5 additional minutes. Keep an eye on them and don't over-cook!

Tasty side dishes include mashed cauliflower (see page 183) and lemon.

Char with roe caviar sauce

Ingredients, serves 4: 1–2 arctic chars (about 1.5 kg (3 lb) in total), 2 tbsp salt (preferably coarse), 1 tsp black pepper, 1 large or 2 small lemons, 100 g (3.5 oz) fresh herbs, preferably thyme and rosemary, 25 g (0.75 oz) butter for frying and to grease the oven dish.

Roe caviar sauce: 100 ml (3.5 fl oz) mayonnaise, 100 ml (3.5 fl oz) crème fraiche, dill, parsley, 1 tbsp lemon juice, dash of pepper, 100 g (3.5 oz) roe, i.e. vendace roe or red lumpfish roe.

Prepare on stove and in oven, 125°C.

Remove the heads from the fish. Using a sharp knife, make angular cuts across the fish. Salt and pepper both inside and outside.

Cut the lemon into slices, chop the herbs and cut 25 g (0.75 oz) of butter into pieces.

Stuff the fish with lemon slices, herbs and butter. Preheat a frying pan and add a generous pat of butter. Brown the fish on both sides to a golden-brown colour.

Place the fish in a buttered oven dish and bake in the oven for about 30 minutes. It's best to use an oven thermometer (place it in the thickest part of the fish). When the temperature reaches 52°C, it's ready.

To make the roe caviar sauce, simply mix all of the ingredients and taste. Excellent!

Poached white fish

Poached fish means that the fish should simmer in water. Fish fillets are poached on the hob. Whole fish should be wrapped in aluminum foil and baked in the oven.

Ingredients, serves 4: about 1 kg (2 lb) headless cod (or other white fish: haddock, pike and pike-perch) or 4 fillets, about 150 g (5.3 oz) each.

Fillets

It's best to use a deep cooking pan.

Add water to the pan until it's half-full. Add fish bouillon, some salt, a few white peppercorns and a laurel leaf. (You can make your own fish bouillon using the fish heads and bones, see page 174)

Boil the water, then reduce the heat to a simmer or remove from the hob.

Place the fillets in the water and let them stand for five minutes. The fish is done when it is white and tender. Do not overcook! The fish will no longer be tender and appealing.

Whole fish

Preheat the oven to 200°C.

Place the cleaned fish on a folded sheet of aluminum foil. Sprinkle with salt and some dill. A few pats of butter will highlight the flavour. Depending on the size of the fish, bake in the oven for 1.5 to 2 hours.

Serving suggestions:

Egg sauce:

Chop three hard-boiled eggs. For convenience, clarify some butter (see page 186). Sprinkle the chopped egg over the fish and top it off with the butter.

For the advanced chef, use some of the fish stock, add cream and slowly simmer to the right consistency. Crème fraiche is also good, but adds a touch of sourness.

With Horse Radish:
Freshly grated horse-radish is sprinkled over the fish. Pour melted butter on top.

With capers, red beets and onions:
Capers, red beets, onions and even lemon wedges with melted butter make a pleasant combination.

Healthier breaded Baltic herring fillets

Ingredients, serves 4: 16 Baltic herring fillets, dill, parsley 2 eggs, 150–200 g (5.3–7 oz) sesame seeds, plenty of butter for frying

Cut the dorsal fin from the herring. Place the fillets with the skin downward, salt and pepper.

Finely chop the parsley and dill. Spread it over the fillets. Place the fillets together with the skin on the outside.

Beat the eggs. Put the sesame seeds onto a flat plate. Turn each fillet, first in the eggs and then in the sesame seeds. Use some pressure so that the seeds stick to the fillets.

Fry them in butter until golden brown, about three minutes on each side.

Tasty side dishes:
Mashed cauliflower (see page 183), flavoured with 1 tsp lemon zest and 1 tsp freshly squeezed lemon.
Lingonberries, raw, stirred with a minimum of sugar (don't add any sugar if you are very sensitive!)

Herring casserole with mustard and cream

Ingredients, serves 4: 1 kg (2 lb) whole or 600 g (1 lb 5 oz) cleaned Baltic herring, 1 leek, 2 tsp herbs (preferably oregano and/or thyme) salt, white pepper, 2 tbsp Dijon mustard or 3 tbsp milder French mustard (unsweetened), 200 ml (7 fl oz) whipping cream, 100 g grated aged cheese, butter for the oven-proof pan.

Preheat the oven to 225°C.

Clean the herring and give them a quick rinse. Place them with the skin-side down on a plate (or a large cutting board with greaseproof paper to avoid absorption of the fish odour).

Finely chop the leeks.

Spread some of the mustard, most of the chopped leeks, salt and pepper and half of the herbs over the fish. Roll the fish and stand them up tightly packed in a buttered oven-proof pan. Distribute the rest of the leeks over the top.

Whisk together the cream with the rest of the mustard, a little salt and some herbs. Sprinkle with cheese.

Bake for about 30 minutes.

Tasty side dishes: mashed broccoli (see page 183)

Pickled Baltic herring

A traditional Scandinavian favourite for Christmas, Easter and Midsummer!

Ingredients, serves 4: 1 kg (2 lb) whole Baltic herring (or 600 g (1 lb 5 oz) cleaned). Marinade: 500 ml (about a pint) water, 125 ml (5 fl oz) triple vinegar (12 %), 1 tbsp salt.

Sauce: 150 ml (5 fl oz) mayonnaise (unsweetened!), 150 ml (5 fl oz) sour cream, 2 tbsp unsweetened, mild mustard, white pepper, 2 garlic cloves (pressed), 1 tsp salt, 100–200 g (3.5–7 oz) finely chopped dill, 50 g (1.75 oz) finely chopped chives.

Clean the fish and remove as many bones as possible. Remove the skin. Briefly rinse the fillets and let them drain. Marinate the fillets for about five hours. Pour off the marinade and carefully drain the fillets, preferably in a strainer. The flesh is now white and firmer.

Mix the sauce ingredients and layer the fillets and sauce in a pot or bowl. There should be sauce on both the bottom and the top. Cover and place in the refrigerator. The dish is ready to serve after two days in the refrigerator. It can also be stored for about five additional days in the refrigerator.

Tasty side dishes:
Boiled egg halves and a few slices of fine aged cheese.

Chicken dishes

When purchasing chicken, the quality of meat is important for your health and for your wallet! Inexpensive, deep-frozen chicken is often injected with water to add weight; the producers charge more because of the added water. Chicken is low in fat, so remember to include rich sauces and side dishes.

Chicken Marengo

Ingredients, serves 4: 1 whole chicken, salt and white pepper, 50 g (1.75 oz) butter, fine soy sauce, rosemary and thyme, 10 baby onions, about 200 g (7 oz) mushrooms, 1 chicken bouillon cube (glutamate-free), 2 tbsp tomato paste, 2 tbsp pressed lemon, about 300 ml (just over half a pint) water.

This is a very old recipe. The dish is said to have originated from the Battle of Marengo, when Napoleon wanted a meal in a big hurry. The cook used what he had at his disposal. Here is a more modern variety.

Cut the chicken into smaller pieces (about 8 pieces). Season it with salt and pepper on all sides. Rub the seasoning in under the skin.

Brown the pieces with a generous pat of butter. Place them in a saucepan, trickle some soy sauce over them and sprinkle with rosemary and thyme.

Sauté the onions and mushrooms and add to the saucepan. Crumble a bouillon cube and add to the mix. Mix the tomato paste with lemon juice and water and pour it in the saucepan.

Cover and simmer the chicken on low heat for about 30 minutes, or until it feels ready. Use a toothpick to check. Juices emerging from the toothpick holes should be completely clear.

Chicken in a clay pot

Ingredients, serves 4: 1 large chicken, 1 tsp salt, 1 tsp lemon, pepper, 1 tsp crushed tarragon, ½ lemon, 1 garlic clove, 10 shallots, 1 red onion, 1 medium-sized carrot, 1 small parsnip, 1 Swedish turnip, 1 small stick of celery, parsley, 100 g (3.5 oz) butter.

Remember to start with a cold oven! Soak the clay pot and lid in cold water for half an hour.

Divide the chicken into pieces and season. Peel the outer layer (zest) from the lemon peel (no white part). Press garlic and lemon over the chicken.

Peel the baby onions and cut the red onion into wedges. Peel the root vegetables and cut them into strips.

Place the vegetables, lemon zest and chicken pieces in the clay pot and top with the butter. Place the wet clay pot in a cold oven and set the oven to 200°C. When the oven temperature has reached 200°C, continue cooking for 45 minutes.

Remove the clay pot and sprinkle the chicken generously with thyme and parsley.

Tasty side dishes:

Creamy gratinated broccoli (see page 183).

Chicken in balsamic vinegar

Ingredients, serves 4: 500 g (1 lb) chicken thigh fillets (juicier and richer than breast fillets), 100 g (3.5 oz) butter, 400 ml (14 fl oz) balsamic vinegar (red wine vinegar also works well), 100 ml (3.5 fl oz) dry white wine, 3 garlic cloves, 1 tbsp tomato paste, salt and white pepper, 3 tbsp chopped fresh herbs (such as tarragon, basil and parsley).

A sauce with vinegar! Strange? There will be a pungent odour during preparation, but after the sauce is reduced, the tangy vinegar taste will be transformed into a bold but delicate flavour.

Divide the chicken fillets into two or three pieces.

Fry them in half of the butter. Cover and let cook through on low heat.

Remove the chicken pieces from the pot and keep them warm.

Chop the garlic. Add vinegar, garlic, wine and tomato paste. Reduce (boil until about ⅓ of the liquid remains) on high heat until the sauce has thickened.

Chop the herbs and add them to the pan.

While stirring, melt the rest of the butter and replace the chicken pieces in the pot with the sauce. Heat before serving.

Tasty side dishes:
A hearty salad containing various types of lettuce, tomatoes and avocado. A generous dab of whisked crème fraiche.

Fillet of chicken with Parma ham, parmesan cheese and tomato salsa

Ingredients, serves 4: 8 thigh fillets (thigh fillets are juicier and fattier than breast fillets and are available at most food stores), 8 sun-dried tomatoes, 8 slices Parma ham (Spanish Serrano ham works just as well), 2 tbsp grated parmesan cheese, fresh basil, about 10 finely chopped olives, salt and white pepper, butter.

Incredible tomato salsa: 4 shallots, 100 g (3.5 oz) butter, 2 garlic cloves, 200 ml (7 fl oz) dry white wine, 200 ml (7 oz) pureed tomatoes, 4 tsp apple cider vinegar (white wine vinegar works well if you do not have apple cider vinegar at home), 200 g (7 oz) chopped fresh basil, 2 tbsp chicken stock, salt and pepper.

Preheat the oven to 200°C.

Unfold the fillets and pound them out thin. Salt and pepper to taste. Add tomato, some parmesan, chopped olives and a couple of basil leaves to one side of the fillet. Fold up the fillet, wrap the package in a slice of Parma ham and place it in a buttered oven-proof pan. For extra flavour, sprinkle some olive oil on the fillets; this will also make them look even more delicious!

Tomato salsa:

Chop the onion and garlic. Quick-fry in half of the butter.

Add the wine and reduce by simmering.

Add the tomatoes, chicken stock, vinegar and chopped basil.

Salt and pepper to taste. For the finishing touch, add the rest of the butter and stir gently.

Tasty side dishes:
A few extra olives, more parmesan cheese to sprinkle on top. Broccoli and/or green salad.

Lazy, spicy au gratin chicken

Ingredients, serves 4: 1 pre-roasted chicken, 1 bell pepper, 300 ml (10.5 fl oz) cream, 1 tbsp freshly grated and pressed ginger, a pinch of chilli, 1 tsp curry, 1 garlic clove, butter for the pan.

Preheat the oven to 225°C.
Bone the chicken and cut into strips. Cut the pepper into strips. Place everything in a buttered oven-proof roasting pan.

Whip the cream until it is frothy. Add the other ingredients. Pour this over the chicken and peppers.

Bake in the oven for about 20 mins.

Tasty side dishes:
Green salad with mayonnaise dressing (see page 187).

Meat dishes

When using lamb, beef and wild game, select high-quality and locally sourced meats if possible.

Cabbage casserole

Ingredients, serves 4: 500 g (1 lb) ground meat (preferably mixed ground pork/beef), about 700 g (1 lb 8 oz) cabbage, 1 leek, 1 yellow onion, at least 1 litre water, 2 tsp salt, 100 g (3.5 oz) butter, 200 ml (7 fl oz) broth (from onion and cabbage), 2 eggs, salt, black or white pepper.

Prepare on the stove and in the oven at 200°C.

Cut away the stem of the cabbage and remove the outer-most leaves if needed; then cut into 1cm-size pieces.

Peel and coarsely chop the onions. Rinse and cut the leeks into coarse strips.

Boil water in a large saucepan. Add the cabbage, leeks and onions and boil with the lid on for 5 minutes. Drain in a strainer; save 200 ml (7 fl oz) of the broth.

Brown the vegetables in a generous amount of butter. Let cool. Coat a baking dish with butter.

Mix 200 ml (7 fl oz) cooled broth with the eggs, salt and pepper. Add the cabbage, onions and ground meat and blend to a smooth, light mixture.

Transfer the mixture to the pan and flatten it out.

Bake the casserole in the middle of the oven for about 1 hour.

Tasty side dishes:
Serve with lingonberries, preferably unsweetened.
Clarified butter.

Tomato salad (sliced tomatoes with finely chopped red onions and dressing).

Feta Hamburger

Ingredients, serves 4: 400 g (14 oz) ground lamb or mixed ground meat, salt and pepper, 4 generous feta cheese slices, crème fraiche, butter (for frying), 1 or 2 slices low-carb bread, fried in butter or grilled with a dab of oil.

For those of you who really miss bread, some grocery stores and Internet sites offer bread with very few carbs (2.7 grams carbs per slice). Toast the slices on a frying pan or grill.

Mix the ground beef as it is with a little salt and pepper.

Form it into patties and fry or grill the burgers about 4 minutes on each side.

Place crème fraiche, the hamburger patty, a slice of feta cheese, more crème fraiche and veggies on a slice of fried or grilled low-carb bread. If desired, top it off with a second slice of bread.

Of course, the burger can be served with no bread and eaten with a knife and fork. A large lettuce leaf is a good substitute for bread.

Wild Game Stew

Ingredients, serves 4: 1 package frozen venison, 1 litre golden chanterelles (fresh, frozen or canned), butter, 2 onions, 10 juniper berries, salt and white pepper, 200 ml (7 fl oz) water with 1 bouillon or broth cube, 250 ml (8.5 fl oz) crème fraiche, parsley.

Quick-fry the mushrooms in plenty of butter and transfer them to a plate.

Quick-fry the venison, a little at a time. Frozen chipped venison works well; it's easy to separate the pieces by hand.

Chop the onions and add them to the meat when it's done. Let the mixture sauté for a moment.

Crush the juniper berries and add them to the pan together with the mushrooms. Salt and pepper to taste. Crumble the bouillon cube and dissolve it in a little water and crème fraîche. Add to the pan. Reduce the heat and simmer for a few minutes. Sprinkle with parsley.

Tasty side dishes :
Green beans and a few lingonberries.

Wiener-schnitzel

Ingredients, serves 4: 4 slices of veal or pork fillets, beaten flat, 2 eggs, 200 g (7 oz) grated parmesan, 100 g (3.5 oz) sesame seeds, 1 lemon, 1 can sardines, 1 small jar of capers, 1 tsp salt, 1 pinch white pepper, butter for frying.

Beat the eggs slightly. Dip fillets in egg.

Put the grated cheese and sesame seeds on a plate. Salt and pepper the cheese mixture.

Press both sides of the egg-coated meat in the cheese and

sesame seed mixture so that it sticks. Dip the fillets once again in more egg.

Fry over low heat with plenty of butter.

Garnish each piece with a slice of lemon, a sardine and a few capers.

Tasty side dishes:

Mashed cauliflower (see page 183), iceberg lettuce with creamy dressing (see page 188). Green peas (rich in carbohydrates, so don't use too many).

Oven-roasted beef brisket

Ingredients, serves 4: 1 kg (2 lb) roast beef, sirloin steak or entrecôte of beef, 1.5 tsp salt, ½ tsp freshly ground pepper, butter for frying.

When roasting cuts of meat in the oven, use low heat and a meat thermometer. This ensures uniform cooking throughout the cut. Even if you like it rare, it will be warm in the middle.

Preheat the oven to 100°C.

Rub the meat with salt and pepper and brown the brisket well on all sides in a frying pan.

Place it in a roasted pan. Insert the meat thermometer in the centre of the meat and place the pan on the middle or lower rack of the oven.

When the thermometer shows 55°C, the meat is rare; at 60°C it's medium-rare. This will take 1.5–2 hours.

Tasty side dishes:
Broccoli au gratin (see page 183), a hearty salad with a tasty dressing, green beans, béarnaise sauce (see page 184).

Lamb sausage (or other high quality sausage) with sauerkraut

Lacto-fermented products are a nutritional treasure; the culture helps preserve the vitamin C and other nutrients. The lactobacilli also add nutrients of their own.

Sauerkraut is a natural probiotic (it contains "friendly" bacteria that are beneficial to the natural flora in the gastrointestinal system, as well as countering the effects of harmful bacteria); an antioxidant (good for the immune system and general health); and reduces the GI for the entire meal.

Sauerkraut promotes good digestion and boosts the immune system.

Olive oil adds extra flavour to sauerkraut (a milder taste and higher fat content). Spices such as rosemary and a pinch of chilli add a special touch.

Bouillon and stock

Basic ingredients for any vegetable broth: 2 litres water, 2 onions, 2 bay leaves, 10 white peppercorns, 2 carrots, 150 g (5.5 oz) celery, thyme, 2.5–3 tsp salt.

Venison stock: Prep time 4–6 hours: 2 kg (4.5 lb) bone and meat scraps, garlic, salt, parsley, rosemary, red wine, cloves, tomato paste, butter, juniper berries, star anise, champignon mushrooms.

Beef stock: prep time 3–4 hours. 2 kg (4.5 lb) bone and meat scraps from beef or veal, leeks, salt, parsley.

Vegetable stock: prep time 2 hours. Parsnip, allspice, rutabaga, cabbage, cauliflower, broccoli.

Fish stock: prep time 20-30 min (low boil). 1–2 kg (2–4.5 lb) heads and bones from raw fish (do not use gills and entrails), white wine, rutabaga, dill, ½ tsp dried crushed tarragon (optional).

Store-bought bouillon cubes, powders and stock can contain hydrogenated fats and glutamate. Homemade bouillon is therefore not only much tastier, but healthier and more rewarding. If you enjoy pottering around the kitchen, you can easily make your own bouillon. It takes some time, but it's not at all difficult. Here's how:

Roast leftover peels, vegetables and meat bones in the oven for half an hour or stir-fry in butter on the stove.

Add water, bring to a boil and let simmer over low heat for 15 minutes–six hours, depending on the contents.

Strain the stock.

If desired, liquefy some of the vegetables and add them to the stock.

Boil over high heat until reduced to half the original volume.

Strain the stock again, preferably through a finer mesh strainer.

It can be frozen in small jars or ice cube trays.

One part stock and one part water provides a fine bouillon.

Soups and hearty salads

Roasted bell pepper soup

Ingredients, serves 4: 6 red bell peppers, deseeded and sliced in two, 2 chopped onions, 3 chopped garlic cloves, 2 tbsp olive oil, 50 g (1.75 oz) butter, 500 ml (just under a pint) vegetable bouillon (preferably homemade, see page 174), 500 ml (just under a pint) cream, 300 g (10.5 oz) coarsely chopped parsley (leaves and stalks), salt and black pepper, crème fraiche, parsley.

Prepare in oven, 225°C, and on the hob.
Place the bell peppers with the skin facing up in an oven pan.

Add the onions and garlic. Trickle olive oil over the vegetables and roast them on the middle rack in the oven for about 25 minutes, or until they are nicely browned.

Remove the peels from the peppers.

Transfer the vegetables to a large saucepan.

Add the vegetable bouillon and parsley and bring to a boil. Boil for 10 minutes without a lid.

Add the butter and use a hand mixer to liquefy the soup.

Serve with a dab of crème fraiche and perhaps some parsley on top.

French fish soup

Ingredients, serves 4: 1 litre (1.75 pints) homemade fish stock (see page 174) or 2 tbsp ready-made fish stock, 1 litre (1.75 pints) water, 750 g (1 lb 10 oz) fresh or frozen fish fillets e.g. pollack, cod and salmon (with only salmon 500 g (1 lb) is enough), 1 carrot, ½ leek, 1 onion, 3 tbsp, cold pressed Canola oil, 50 g (1.75 oz) butter, 2 garlic cloves, 1 packet saffron, 3 tomatoes, 300 ml (10.5 fl oz) cream, 250 g (9 oz) shelled shrimp, basil, chilli pepper (if you like it hot), salt and pepper, chives.

Bring the water to a boil and scald the tomatoes for a minute or so. Rinse the tomatoes with cold water, make a cut and pull off the skins.

Peel the vegetables and cut them into thin strips. Carefully fry them on low heat in a large saucepan with butter.

Chop the garlic and add it to the saffron.

Add the fish stock (homemade or store-bought) and water; then add the peeled tomatoes.

Stir in the cream and let boil for 10 minutes.

Shell the shrimp. Cut the fish into large pieces and place in the saucepan. Add the largest pieces first. Simmer for about five minutes. Avoid vigorous boiling – the fish will then become dry and unappealing. Salt and pepper to taste.

Chop the chives and basil leaves and sprinkle them on top together with the shrimp.

Tasty side dishes:
A dab of rouille or aioli (see page 187).

Gazpacho

Spanish national dish. Serve cold!

Ingredients, serves 4: 4 tomatoes, 1 cucumber, 1 onion, 1 green bell pepper, 1.5 tbsp vegetable stock (preferably home-made, see page 174), 4 tbsp olive oil, 1 tbsp pressed lemon, a few drops of Tabasco, black pepper, salt if needed, about 500 ml (just under a pint) water, 2 garlic cloves.

Rinse and cut into pieces 3 tomatoes, ⅔ of the cucumber and the bell pepper.

Peel the onion and cut it into pieces. Set aside half of the bell pepper and transfer the rest of the vegetables to a blender. Blend the vegetables into a purée (about 30 seconds).

Mix the purée and the vegetable stock together with the oil, lemon juice, Tabasco, pepper and salt (if needed). Add water to taste.

Finely chop the rest of the vegetables and add them to the soup together with pressed garlic.

Tasty side dishes :
Crispy bacon slices.

Tuscan chick pea soup

Ingredients, serves 4: 2 cans of chick peas, 500 ml (just under a pint) water, 500 ml (just under a pint) cream, some concentrated or homemade stock, 1 sprig rosemary butter, 1 slice bacon.

Mash most of the beans and boil together with the water, the stock and the bacon slice for about 10 minutes.

Heat the rosemary leaves in some butter. When they have softened, add them to the soup together with the whole chick peas.

Tasty side dishes:
Mix 2 tbsp olive oil and 2 tbsp balsamic vinegar and trickle on top.

Crispy bacon.

Niçoise Salad

Ingredients, serves 4: 4 portions, 1 can tuna in oil, 150 g (5.5 oz) high-fat cheese, 1 can green beans, 1 thinly-sliced red onion, 4 tomatoes, 10 black olives, 4 hard-boiled eggs, 2 tbsp capers or 1 small can sardines, 1 lemon, olive oil.

The traditional Niçoise salad contains potatoes, but as carb-sensitive eaters, we will eliminate those from the recipe. We will use more eggs and cheese instead.

Divide the tuna into pieces with a fork.

Strain the brine from the beans and olives.

Slice the tomatoes.

Gently mix everything in a bowl so that it doesn't get mashed together; alternatively, serve each ingredient separately and let everyone create their own salad.

Garnish with egg and lemon slices.

Caesar salad with chicken

Ingredients, serves 4: 3–4 chicken fillets (fried in butter), 1 head of lettuce, preferably Romaine lettuce, 1 egg, 1 tbsp white wine vinegar, 3 sardines, 1 tsp light Dijon mustard, salt, black pepper, 1 small garlic clove, about 100 ml (3.5 fl oz) cold-pressed canola oil at room temperature, 4 tbsp freshly grated parmesan,

Rinse the lettuce thoroughly and refrigerate in a plastic bag for one hour.

To make the sauce: boil the egg for 2 minutes, remove it and cool it quickly under cold running water. Scoop out the egg yolk and put it in a blender or salad bowl. Add the vinegar, mustard and sardines (mash the sardines with a fork if you're using a salad bowl)

Add salt, pepper and pressed garlic. Mix in the bowl or in the blender. Add the oil in a thin stream while mixing. Mix in the parmesan cheese.

Slice the butter-fried chicken fillets in whatever size pieces you prefer and distribute them over the salad.

Tasty side dishes:
Stir-fried Savoy cabbage with bacon, apple and nuts

Tasty side dishes

Stir-fried savoy cabbage with bacon, apple and nuts

4 portions: 50 g bacon, 1/2 head Savoy cabbage, 1 (sour) apple, 2 dl crème fraiche, 1/2 lemon, 1 dl roasted nuts, preferably walnuts, butter for frying, flake salt.

Sauté the bacon and cabbage in butter until it starts to brown; use a wok or frying pan.

Transfer the cabbage mixture to a plate.

Cut the apples into wedges, quickly stir fry them in butter; stir in the cabbage and crème fraîche and top it off with some pressed lemon juice.

Garnish with nuts and a few pinches of salt.

Helpful hints
Roast the nuts (walnuts) to a golden brown in the oven at 175°C for 5–10 minutes.

Ratatouille

4 portions: 3 large onions, 4 bell peppers, 1 zucchini, 1 small aubergine, 2 tbsp olive oil, 50 g butter, 1 can all tomatoes, 3

garlic cloves, basil, thyme, 1 laurel leaf, salt, a bit of white pepper.

Rinse, peel and cut all of the vegetables into pieces as desired (except garlic and tomatoes). Sauté them in a saucepan with the oil and butter.

Peel and finely chop the garlic. Add the garlic and canned tomatoes to the saucepan. Boil for 15 minutes. Stir occasionally.

Add the spices and boil without a lid for 20 minutes until it thickens. Stir occasionally.

Add salt and pepper to taste (Add a few pats of butter just before serving.)

Gratinated aubergine

4 portions: 2 aubergine, 3 large onions, 2 large chopped garlic cloves, 1 medium zucchini, 2 tsp thyme, 4 medium tomatoes, 1 dl whipping cream, 2 tsp French mustard, 1 dl grated aged cheese, butter for frying.

Prepare on stove and in oven, 250° C.

Peel the aubergines and slice them into thin slices (about ½ cm). Fry them lightly in butter. Place them on a platter.

Chop the onion and garlic and sauté them on low heat for 7 minutes.

Slice the zucchini. Sauté them on low heat in butter and some thyme for about 5 minutes.

Layer the eggplant slices in a large oven pan.

Cover with onions, then zucchini slices and lastly the sliced tomato.

Mix the mustard with the cream and pour the mixture over the vegetables.

Bake in the oven for about 50 minutes. Distribute the cheese on top, and return the pan to the oven for an additional 10 minutes.

Mashed cauliflower and/or broccoli

4 portions: 1 large cauliflower (or 2 large heads of broccoli) or half cauliflower and half broccoli, 2 dl whipping cream, 1 tsp salt, 1 pinch ground white pepper (a pinch of nutmeg), 2 tsp (or more) butter.

Smooth, tasty and a perfect alternative to carbohydrate-rich mashed potatoes.

Trim the cauliflower or broccoli and divide it into bouquets.

Boil the cabbage in cream in a covered, thick-bottomed saucepan for 5–10 minutes or until soft.

Stir occasionally to prevent the cream from burning.

Remove the lid and boil until most of the liquid has evaporated.

Remove from heat and mix with an electric mixer or blender. Add butter, salt and pepper.

Gratinated broccoli

4 portions: 2 large heads of fresh (or an equal amount of frozen) broccoli, 2 dl cream, 2 dl crème fraiche, 2 eggs, 200 g gorgonzola, salt and pepper.

Cut the entire broccoli into pieces and preboil until it begins to soften.

Mix the cream, crème fraîche and eggs and season with salt and pepper.

Place the hot broccoli in an oven pan and pour the cream mixture on top.

Top with crumbled Gorgonzola and bake in the oven until the cream mixture thickens and the surface is golden-brown.

Béarnaise sauce

4–5 portions: 150 g butter, 2 tbsp white wine vinegar, 1 tbsp fresh or 2 tsp dried tarragon, 2 tbsp chopped shallots (or yellow onion), 1 sprig parsley, 2 tbsp water, 3 egg yolks, salt and white pepper. Note!! All ingredients should be at room temperature.

Prepare with a food processor and saucepan.

Peel and coarsely chop the onions. Boil the onions, parsley sprig, vinegar and crushed tarragon in a small saucepan for a few minutes or until most of the liquid has evaporated.

Add 2 tbsp water and mix.

Remove the parsley sprig and pour the vinegar mixture into the food processor.

Add the egg yolks and start the processor for a few seconds.

Melt the butter on low heat; raise the heat towards the end. The butter should be hot (but not browned).

Turn on the food processor and slowly pour a thin stream of hot butter through the opening while the machine is running.

Season with white pepper and salt to taste.

Heat the sauce on the stovetop, but do not boil! This will curdle the sauce.

Season the butter with salt, mustard powder, garlic, thyme, paprika powder, chili powder, tarragon, lemon and finely chopped onion.

Melt the butter and whisk it to a fine sauce.

Seasoned butter

Seasoned butter is easy to prepare and is an excellent condiment that enhances the flavor of and increases fat content with steak, pork chops, meat loaf and other dishes that often are too lean.

Seasoning tips: Parsley, herbs, horseradish, chili, grated sharp cheese, pepper, lemon, lime, orange.

4 portions: 1 tsp concentrated veal stock, 1/2 dl water, 2.5 dl sour cream, 2 tbsp Worcestershire sauce, salt & pepper.

Mix all of the ingredients and heat carefully.

Remoulade sauce

4 portions: 1 dl mayonnaise, 2 dl crème fraiche, 1 tbsp curry, 2 tbsp horseradish, 1 dl chopped gherkins, 1 small leek, salt and pepper, some lemon juice.

Chop the gherkin; thoroughly rinse the leek inside and out and cut into thin slices. Mix all of the ingredients in a bowl and season with salt, pepper and some lemon juice.

Serve with fried fish or roast beef.

Butter sauce (Sooo good!)

4 portions: 2 finely chopped baby onions (preferably shallots), 1 dl dry white wine, 2 tbsp white wine vinegar, 1 parsley sprig, 5 white pepper corns, 2 tbsp whipping cream, 100 g butter at room temperature, salt and pepper.

Chop the onions and mix all of the ingredients except for butter and cream in a saucepan.

Boil until only a couple of tablespoons of liquid remain, filter, strain off the fluid and pour it back into the saucepan.

Add cream and bring to a boil.

Remove the saucepan from heat and whisk in the butter a dab at a time. Heat the sauce carefully occasionally as required, but do not boil! Salt and pepper to taste.

Serving suggestion
1 tbsp vendace roe and 1 tbsp finely chopped chive (great with fish).

1 tbsp finely grated horseradish (good with meat and fish), 1 tbsp cognac or calvados (excellent with meat and fish). 1 tbsp finely chopped fresh tarragon (tasty with everything).

Grated rind of 1 lime and a smidgen of finely chopped red chili (goes with poultry and fish).

Clarified butter
Melt the butter. Skim off the froth, then carefully pour the butter into another container, leaving the white milk solids at the bottom of the saucepan.

Serve the clarified butter with salmon, herring and most anything.

Mayonnaise

Note! Ingredients should be at room temperature.

3 dl, 2 egg yolks, 1 tbsp freshly pressed lemon, 1/2 tsp French mustard, 2 dl cold-pressed canola oil or mild olive oil

Mix the egg yolks, lemon juice and mustard and whisk together or use a blender or food processor to blend for a few seconds.

Continue mixing and slowly drip the oil into the mixture. Whisk until the mayonnaise has thickened. Keep cold in a tightly closed container. Mayonnaise can be stored up to one week in the refrigerator.

Aioli

Season the mayonnaise with 2 pressed garlic cloves.

Rouille

Exclude the mustard from the mayonnaise recipe and season with 1 g saffron, 2 pressed garlic cloves and 1 teaspoon cayenne pepper.

Tzatziki

1 liter Turkish yoghurt, 1 cucumber salt, 3 garlic cloves, 2 tbsp olive oil

Peel and coarsely shred the cucumber.

Put cucumber in a strainer and sprinkle some salt over it. Let stand for half an hour. The salt will help draw water out of the cucumber.

Press the shredded cucumber with a spoon to remove the water. Mix the yogurt and cucumber, add the pressed garlic and stir in olive oil.

Creamy dressing

2 dl cream, juice and finely grated rind of 1 lemon, salt and pepper

Mix the cream and lemon until the cream thickens a bit. Season with salt and pepper.

A wonderfully fresh and smooth dressing that perfectly complements crispy lettuce.

Ruccola is a popular favorite, dill and parsley with fish, or large, crispy lettuce leaves with a grilled steak.

Afterword

I've been on a low-carb diet since the autumn of 2003. At the time of writing, it's March 2011. We often hear that there's no way to predict the long-term effects of eating as few carbo-hydrates as I do. I find this quite amusing. We know with cer-tainty that the official dietary recommendations for diabetics lead to a debilitating situation that is so commonplace that we have even named it "the natural course of events". Those responsible for the current "official" (and poor) dietary advice may find comfort in the notion that it's not "harmful"; these people claim that it is simply "natural" for diabetics to have their feet amputated after a certain time – if they live long enough.

THE SCANDINAVIAN DIET, on the other hand, contains only small amounts of the things that destroy a diabetic's body, making it an unlikely cause of any negative side effects. In the short-term, all diabetics will experience an almost immediate improvement in their blood sugar values. In the long-term, no negative effects of THE SCANDINAVIAN DIET have yet been reported.

To summarise their conclusion, as strange as it may seem; the certainty of ill health is preferable to uncertainty.

Although it has long been held that diabetics have a life expectancy about ten years shorter than the average – and significantly more for Type 1 diabetics – over the last decades there has been a drastic improvement, with over 51.5% now living longer. All the same, there is plenty of room for improvement of the long-term survival rate. Type 2 diabetics will feel much better if they stop provoking their bodies with high-carb intake and the resulting increase of their blood sugar and insulin levels. Years of quality time can be added to their lives.

I'm dumbfounded by the fact that entire groups of experts have had such a difficult time recognising this connection. The diabetic's problem is that he or she cannot cope with sugar and starch. These substances cause injury to the body. What could be simpler than avoiding foods that contain sugar and starch? We actually do hear that refined sugar is bad, but I venture to say that other foods, such as bread and pasta, are even more dangerous.

The most recent review of diabetes treatment in Sweden resulted in a most astounding conclusion: there is no scientific basis for today's recommendations. For some reason, modern and smaller-scale studies on diabetes and diet were ignored, resulting in the conclusion that there isn't any scientific basis for the advice I offer in this book either. That leaves us trapped between a rock and a hard place. The old advice is only thought to be sound because it has been around longer, despite the fact that it is equally unsupported by scientific evidence. This is a striking example of how medical logic can work.

My position is that dietary advice shouldn't even be offered, because we know too little. What we (diabetics) should do is to try things and see ourselves how it works for us. It needn't be anything dramatic. Measure your blood sugar level after a "recommended" breakfast and after a breakfast recommended in this book (bacon and eggs). You won't be relying on second- or third-hand information, but on authentic first-hand information. You'll find out exactly what's happening to you! Isn't that great? If you're taking insulin, you'll need to monitor your blood sugar carefully, so that it doesn't sink too low after a breakfast according to THE SCANDINAVIAN DIET. Eating this way will help you get better without needles, so insulin administration may cause your blood sugar level to sink dangerously low.

If you really stick to THE SCANDINAVIAN DIET, you may be able to eliminate all the pills and needles and never worry about the risk of low blood sugar. THE SCANDINAVIAN DIET gives your body a chance to maintain a comfortable and healthy level.

Another bonus of LCHF (low-carb high fat) for the type 2 diabetic is the opportunity to lose weight. The body will generally "normalise" by itself on THE SCANDINAVIAN DIET. Yet another bonus is that you will be able to eat really tasty food, with real butter and real cream. Recent studies indicate that salt is not the villain it has been made out to be, so you now have at your disposal the professional chef's arsenal of salt, butter and cream to prepare delicious meals!

Swedish medical authorities have confirmed that THE SCANDINAVIAN DIET, as a treatment for obesity and diabetes, is consistent with current scientific understanding and proven experience. For those of you longing to eat real food again, wait no longer. Go for it and start enjoying your new life!

Acknowledgements

I would like to express my sincere gratitude to all those who provided valuable support and advice. Among them: Uffe Ravnskov, Erik Edlund, Bo Zackrisson och Karl Arfors.

At the time of writing, the symposium is available at mms://wmedia.it.su.se/kv/kva081120.wmv

More information in "Fear of Fat", Optimal Publishing

Läkartidningen 2008-10-21: *Kan man lita på kliniska studier,* Fredrik Hedlund, freelance journalist

Lesser LI, Ebbeling CB, Goozner M, Wypij D, Ludwig DS (2007) Relationship between Funding Source and Conclusion among Nutrition-Related Scientific Articles. PLoS Med 4 (1): e5. Doi:10. 1371/journal.pmed.0040005

Let me hold your hand trough the whole process.
Take a look at our 6 weeks', step by step, coaching
program that will guide you through The Scandinavian Diet
in a safe, easy and comfortable way! I will teach you all the
Proven Techniques and make sure YOU learn how to eat in
a healthy way and really start enjoying YOUR LIFE! I will
guide YOU, encourage YOU and support YOU every step
of the way!

Lose Your Excess Fat ... Get Your Optimal Health!
Without Ever Having To Feel Hungry Again!

Go to our web page www.scandinaviandiet.co.uk or ring
01614082979 for more information and allow me to help
you!

Warmly,
Victoria Aase
Licensed Scandinavian Diet Coach

LOSE WEIGHT BY EATING
February 2012

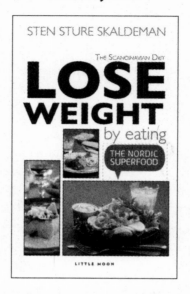

From 150 to 80 kilos! Welcome to LOSE WEIGHT BY EATING, your first step on the road back to slimness and full health.

Whether you are mildly overweight or grossly obese, Sten Skaldeman has the answer.

By choosing the right foods and adopting a few simple principles, Sten Skaldeman shows you how you can, quite literally, lose weight without ever having to starve yourselves again.

In LOSE WEIGHT BY EATING, Sten Skaldeman leads you back toward the diet mankind is adapted to. By choosing these foods, you can, quite literally, lose weight without ever having to starve yourself again.

THE SCANDINAVIAN DIET
February 2012

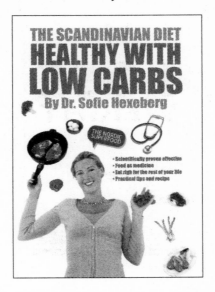

"Books like THE SCANDINAVIAN DIET are essential reading if you want to learn how to live a truly happy, healthy life."

Barry Groves,
Author of *Trick and Treat: How Healthy Eating is Making Us Ill*

In THE SCANDINAVIAN DIET, Dr Sofie Hexeberg shows you how you can protect yourself from obesity, heart disease, diabetes, and all sort of other conditions – not through drugs, but by simple changes in your diet.

Exhaustively researched and based on close clinical studies, THE SCANDINAVIAN DIET is a programme few of us – no matter how overweight or unwell we are – can afford to ignore.